Communication Skills in Practice

Sl THE LC ᵒS
M

of related interest

Cognitive Behaviour Therapy in Primary Care
Richard France and Meredith Robson
1 85302 410 4

Staff Supervision in a Turbulent Environment
Managing Process and Task in Front-line Services
Lynette Hughes and Paul Pengelly
1 85302 327 2

Collaboration in Health and Welfare
Working with Difference
Ann Loxley
1 85302 394 9

Communication Skills in Practice
A Practical Guide for Health Professionals

Diana Williams

Jessica Kingsley Publishers
London and Bristol, Pennsylvania

The right of Diana Williams to be identified as author of this work has been asserted by her in accordance with the Copyright, Designs and Patents Act 1988.

First published in the United Kingdom in 1997 by
Jessica Kingsley Publishers Ltd
116 Pentonville Road
London N1 9JB, England
and
1900 Frost Road, Suite 101
Bristol, PA 19007, U S A

Copyright © 1997 Diana Williams

Library of Congress Cataloging in Publication Data
Williams, Diana, 1957–
Communication skills in practice : a practical guide for health
professionals / Diana Williams.
p.   cm.
Includes bibliographical references and index.
ISBN 1-85302-232-2 (PB)
1. Communication in medicine.   2. Interpersonal communication.
I. Title.
[DNLM: 1. Communication. 2. Interpersonal Relations.   W62 W722c
1996]
R118.W54   1996
610.69'6--dc20
DNLM/DLC
for Library of Congress   96-11245
                                                                  CIP

British Library Cataloguing in Publication Data
Williams, Diana
Communication skills in practice : a practical guide for
health professionals
1. Communication in human services 2. Medical personnel and
patient 3. Public health – Great Britain
I. Title
362.1'014

ISBN 1-85302-232-2

Printed and Bound in Great Britain by
Athenaeum Press, Gateshead, Tyne and Wear

Contents

Acknowledgements ix

Introduction 1

Part One: Communication Skills 3

1 Non-Verbal Communication 6
Proximity 6
Touch 7
Eye-contact and eye-gaze 9
Facial expression 10
Gesture 12
Body posture 14
Head movements 15

2 Paralinguistic Features of Communication 17
Quality of voice 17
Volume 17
Intonation and pitch 18
Rate of speech 19
Tone of voice 19
Conversational oil 20

3 Verbal Communication 21
What makes a good verbal communicator? 21
Advanced verbal skills relevant to professionals 21

Part Two: Interviews 29

4 Purpose of Interviews 33

5 Scene Setting 35

6 Gathering Information 42

7 Involving the Interviewee 55

8 Completing the Interview 64

9 Dealing with Difficult Situations 69

10 Working with Interpreters 75

11 Interviewing Skills in Context 86
11.1 Clinical Interviews 86
11.2 Appraisal Interviews 118
11.3 Recruitment Interviews 133
11.4 Grievance and Disciplinary Interviews 159
11.5 Interviews with the Media 166

Part Three: Professional Meetings 173

12 Preparation 176

13 Communication Roles 183

14 Presenting Self 203

15 Meetings Skills in Context 208
15.1 Business Meetings 208
15.2 Multi-disciplinary Teams 213
15.3 Case Conferences 223
15.4 Committees 225
15.5 Working Parties 232

Part Four: Presentation Skills 235

16 Preparation 239

17 Effective Use of Voice 253

18 Delivering Content 280

19 Establishing Rapport with the Audience 288

20 Using Non-Verbal Communication 294

21 Effective Use of Audio Visual Aids 301

22 Presentation Skills in Context 319

22.1 Client/Carer Workshops 333

22.2 Presentations to other Professionals 339

22.3 Lectures 339

22.4 Selling your Service 351

22.5 Presenting your Research 357

References 368

Subject Index 375
Author Index 381

List of Tables

Table 2.1   Self-evaluation of appraisal objectives   130
Table 4.1   Table of common audio-visual aids and their specific
             features   304

List of Figures

Figure 2.1 (a) (b) (c) Types of seating arrangements used in interviews   87/88
Figure 3.1   Example of the joint objectives of a speech therapist and
              specialist health visitor   218
Figure 3.2   Example of the skills and expertise shared between
              a speech therapist and a specialist health visitor   219
Figure 3.3   Example of shared management plan   220
Figure 4.1   An example of a brainstorm on the topic of 'stopping
              smoking'   243
Figure 4.2   Prioritising points from a spider's web   243
Figure 4.3   Diagram showing the lungs and diaphragm   255
Figure 4.4   The Vocal Tract   257
Figure 4.5   Cross section of the vocal folds showing the opening
              and closing phases   258
Figure 4.6   Example of an evaluation form   346
Figure 4.7   Example of an evaluation form   347
Figure 4.8   Example of an evaluation form   348
Figure 4.9   Vertical bar chart   360
Figure 4.10 Horizontal bar chart   360
Figure 4.11 Multiple bar chart   361
Figure 4.12 Proportional bar chart   362
Figure 4.13 Pie chart   363
Figure 4.14 Line chart   364

Acknowledgements

There are many people who have offered their time, support and encouragement to this project. I would particularly like to thank Robert Freeburn, Stephanie Martin and David Carey for their interest and advice regarding the voice section of this book. (A special thank you to David for allowing me to give my own voice a workout, whilst researching the book.) A big thank you and large hugs to Eugene Doyen, Shemiu Idowu and Roger West for their patience, support and advice; and for their emergency first aid for my numerous computer problems. My gratitude for the valuable comments and suggestions from Ruth Herbert and Brian Haines who read through parts of the draft. I would also like to acknowledge the contributions of John Furze, Pat Honeysett, Annette Maczka and Sally Williams. A special thanks to Jessica Kingsley for her patience and forbearance. Finally, but not least, I would like to express my appreciation to all my former colleagues at the Central School of Speech and Drama.

Special Notes

Please note that he or she is used interchangeably in the text. This is an attempt to avoid any bias arising from the use of one gender.

Introduction

The health professional is required to develop and maintain a high level of interpersonal communication. The nature of health care demands expertise in interviewing, explaining, giving instructions and advising. The development of these professional skills is initiated during the individual's training in the theoretical and practical aspects of their particular discipline. The student is exposed to models of good practice in the management and care of the client during practical placements. In addition, many courses now include a teaching module specifically on communication skills.

The transition from student to clinician brings new communicative demands for the individual. She will continue to extend and elaborate her clinical skills. She must also fulfil the role of the 'professional' and the 'team member'. This will involve attendance at staff meetings and participation in performance review – activities in which individuals rarely receive training.

Clinicians who choose to make the move into management will need to acquire the appropriate skills to deal effectively with staff and resources. They will be faced with a number of situations that require excellent interpersonal skills. These range from appraisal and recruitment interviews to more serious matters such as disciplinary hearings.

This book provides the health professional with practical guidance in developing and maintaining effective communication skills. It covers a wide range of both clinical and professional situations, and these are grouped under the three areas of interviewing, professional meetings and presentations. It is intended for use by a variety of health care workers that include therapists, health visitors, general practitioners, and nurses. Some sections are pertinent to the student, whereas others will help the practitioner meet the varied demands placed on the professional.

The book is divided into four sections. The first section provides the reader with a comprehensive description of the verbal and non-verbal behaviours involved in communication. These definitions form a common terminology for later sections, which deal with a variety of clinical and professional contexts. The main part of each section provides general information on skills and processes. These skills are then applied to specific contexts.

How to Use the Book

The book is designed to give the reader easy access to information. A breakdown of topic areas is provided at the beginning of each part, so that the reader can quickly identify sections of interest.

Alternatively, the reader can refer to the summary points at the end of each chapter. These provide a brief guide to the content of each subsection.

PART ONE

Communication Skills

1. ## Non-Verbal Communication
   Proximity
   Touch
   Eye-Contact and Eye-Gaze
   Facial Expression
   Gesture
   Body Posture
   Head Movements

2. ## Paralinguistic Features of Communication
   Quality of Voice
   Volume
   Intonation and Pitch
   Rate of Speech
   Tone of Voice
   Conversational Oil

3. ## Verbal Communication
   What Makes a Good Verbal Communicator?
   Advanced Verbal Skills Relevant to Professionals

Communication Skills – A Definition

Communication skills have been traditionally classified into verbal and non-verbal behaviours. This section offers a comprehensive description of these behaviours. It is intended to stimulate the reader's interest and act as an introduction to the study of communication. There are three main parts covering non-verbal communication, paralinguistic features of communication and verbal communication. The reader will find it helpful to refer to this section for definitions of terms used within the main body of the book.

Non-verbal communication

Non-verbal communication, or as it is more popularly known, body language, refers to those movements and positions of the head, limbs and body that convey meaning. These behaviours serve several functions, which can be summarised as:

- giving information
- seeking information
- expressing emotions
- communicating interpersonal attitudes (e.g. warmth, dominance, liking)
- establishing and maintaining relationships
- regulating social interaction.

This section looks at specific behaviours and examines their role in relation to these different functions. They include:

- proximity
- touch
- eye-contact and eye-gaze
- facial expression
- gesture
- body posture
- head movements.

The reader is reminded that although these behaviours are presented in isolation they should not be considered as discrete entities. For one thing they often occur simultaneously – for example, interest is expressed through facial expression and posture at the same time. One behaviour will also affect another. So, the act of making a gesture automatically results in a change of posture.

Paralinguistic features of communication

This section looks at the paralinguistic or vocal aspects of our communication. Paralinguistic features include:

- quality of voice
- volume
- intonation and pitch
- rate of speech
- conversational oil
- tone of voice.

Like non-verbal communication, they express emotions and convey information about interpersonal attitudes. Some aspects like tone, intonation and pitch can alter meaning. Variation of these dimensions can enliven the spoken word, and are often used to great effect by presenters, actors and other public speakers.

Verbal communication

What makes a good verbal communicator?

This section gives a brief summary of the different aspects of verbal language. This is followed by a discussion of the qualities and characteristics of an effective communicator.

Advanced verbal skills relevant to professionals

This section looks at some of the reasons that health professionals need advanced verbal skills.

1

Non-Verbal Communication

Proximity

Proximity refers to the distance participants maintain between themselves during social encounters. Hall (1966) proposed that it was possible to classify this space according to the purpose of the encounter. He identified four zones – intimate; personal; social or consultative; and public.

An intimate zone is a distance of 18 inches (45cm) or less. We only choose to get this close to people with whom we have a loving or intimate relationship. Each of us also has a personal space of between 18 inches and 4 feet (45cm–1.2m). We tend to keep this distance when we are talking to friends or engaged in an informal encounter. All of us will be familiar with the feeling of discomfort caused when someone breaks the rules by invading our personal space. This is even more threatening if a person trespasses into our intimate zone.

Most health professionals maintain a social or consultative distance of between 4 feet and 12 feet (1.2m–3.6m). However, they are members of one of the few professions where it is legitimate to enter not only the personal zone, but the intimate one as well. Diagnosis and treatment often involves close physical contact with the client.

Distances greater than 12 feet (3.6m) are usually employed by public speakers, as a way of separating themselves from the audience. They may also try to achieve a difference in height, by raising themselves on a platform for example. Both distance and height increase the likelihood that all members of the audience will be able to see them.

We can see from Hall's classification that distance is also closely linked to the relationship between the participants. People who like each other tend to stand or sit closer. Distance also tells us about the relationship between people in terms of status. Those who are similar in rank or position maintain closer proximity than those who have an unequal relationship (Zahn 1991).

Sometimes these rules about personal space are broken, because the context of a social encounter also has an effect on the distance that individuals adopt. For instance, close bodily contact is tolerated between two strangers on a crowded train, but would seem inappropriate and unwelcome if these individuals were alone in an empty compartment. Dancing is another example where it is acceptable for relative strangers to dance very close.

Conventions about proximity also vary between cultures (Noesjirwan 1978), and seem to be linked with how much bodily contact is the social norm. People who touch more, tend to stand closer. Distance may vary then because of the context, the role that we adopt, or our cultural background.

Touch

Touch is a powerful form of communication despite its relative lack of sophistication when compared with other non-verbal signals. It is associated with strong emotions at both ends of the spectrum, such as love, sexual attraction and aggression. The intimacy of touch is reflected by the strict codes that govern its use. These rules determine the amount of touch, the type of touch, who we touch and where we touch each other. These rules are closely related to the relationship between people, and the context in which touch is being used.

Each society has its set of rules about bodily contact. They also place different interpretations on touch from one culture to another. So a continental kiss on both cheeks is acceptable between heterosexual men in Greece, but not in England. Some of these differences seem to be related to whether people are from a contact or non-contact culture. A study by Jourard (1966) showed that people varied in the amount and type of touch they used with each other. This was related to their cultural background. So Greek people belong to a contact culture, and the English to a non-contact culture.

Touch is probably the most important non-verbal behaviour for the health professional, because of its function in diagnosis and treatment. There are many examples of its role in health care. Touch, like the other senses of the body, is essential to the clinical examination. For example, a doctor will feel the size, shape and location of a lump. Touch is also a treatment medium. Physiotherapists and osteopaths need to manipulate their clients.

The health professional will also be monitoring the clients response to touch. The way in which a client reacts to touch is significant. For instance, a loss of sensation indicates a disturbance to the nervous system; a response of pain to touch is symptomatic of many diseases. For the health professional touch is an integral part of their clinical procedures.

The fact that touch is also a form of communication is sometimes forgotten, and sometimes deliberately avoided in the health care context. Touch is restricted to a purely clinical role. This may be a response to the difficulty of crossing the normal social boundaries about whom we touch and where we touch them. However, the health professional can make considerable use of touch as another way of communicating with the client. For some of these clients touch is the only channel of communication. For example, the client who has difficulty in understanding following a stroke; or the very young infant.

Here are some thoughts about the positive aspects of touch:

- Touch is important for our well-being
- Touch helps us relax
- Touch makes us feel safe
- Touch reassures
- Touch heals
- Touch offers comfort
- Touch is warmth
- Touch is togetherness.

Touch communicates:

- I care
- I can help
- I am concerned about you
- I feel sad too
- I am happy for you
- I will miss you.

Some clients may have lost their ability to use the spoken word, for example the client who has had a laryngectomy. Others, like the elderly client who suffers from dementia, may have difficulty putting their thoughts into words.

What are these clients trying to say to us through touch?

- I trust you
- I am afraid
- I need you
- I am grateful
- I feel sad

- I am lonely
- I feel frightened
- I like you.

The health professional uses many different types of touch that help and support the client:

- cradling an infant
- holding hands
- an arm around the shoulder
- a hug
- smoothing a brow
- lifting
- shaking a hand
- linking arms to steady somebody's gait.

What types of touch do you use with your clients?

Touch evokes powerful reactions; and not everyone likes to be touched. They may feel embarrassed, uncomfortable or even threatened. You will be able to make some predictions about their response to touch from their cultural background and gender. Use your instincts to judge what seems comfortable for them.

Eye-contact or eye-gaze

Eye-contact and eye-gaze are terms that people employ to describe a variety of gaze patterns. These include how often and for how long a person looks at someone else and whether that gaze is returned. Looking is a form of communication, as well as a channel for collecting information. We need to look at someone to get feedback and to monitor their non-verbal behaviour.

Eye-gaze also communicates information about our attitudes to people (Argyle and Cook 1976). For centuries, poets, artists and musicians have recognised the role of eye-contact in attraction. Research has confirmed this strong link between looking and liking (Argyle and Dean 1965). We look more at people we like. The reverse of this is when too much looking becomes uncomfortable and threatening. A stare is hostile, and often precedes aggressive behaviour.

Gaze also has a role in regulating and controlling the flow of communication. It is an important signal for turn-taking in conversation. When a person finishes what she wants to say, she will look at the other person. The listener perceives this as a cue that it is their turn to speak. If the speaker wants to pause but is not yet ready to relinquish the speaker role, she will look away.

Research has found that the amount people look at each other during conversation is different depending on whether they are speaking or listening. The listener looks more at the speaker and for longer amounts of time, than *vice versa* (Kleinke 1986). The speaker's gaze is more intermittent, with the amount of eye-gaze decreasing as the complexity of the material increases (Gahagan 1975). Periods of mutual gaze tend to be short lived.

The reason listeners spend a lot of time looking is linked to its function as a social reinforcer. One way of showing that we are paying attention is to look at the other person. The old joke about the husband that hides behind his newspaper at breakfast illustrates the frustration created by a lack of eye-contact. By looking we also have the opportunity to observe the other person. This is why the speaker will also glance at the listener. They want to get feedback on how the other person is reacting to their message.

The amount of eye-gaze used by people varies between cultures. People tend to look more if they are from a culture that allows a lot of bodily contact during social encounters (Watson 1970). There are also rules and conventions about the use of gaze. Many cultures discourage eye-contact. The gender of the participants seems to be an influencing factor in these rules. For instance in India it is viewed as provocative for a woman to look a man in the eyes (L'Armand 1984).

Despite these differences Watson found that different patterns of gaze were interpreted in a similar way. Too much gaze was regarded as threatening or superior, whereas too little was viewed as inattentive or insincere.

Individuals may change their normal gaze patterns if they suffer any disturbance of mood. Sad or depressed people tend to look less and to look down. Gaze also tends to be averted in people with mental health problems. These characteristics are obviously of significance to the health professional.

Facial expression

The photofit of the wanted criminal or missing person is incomplete without a portrayal of the facial features. Physical variations of size, shape and colour, and the use of idiosyncratic expressions help to form individual identities. These features are often interpreted, although not always accurately, as representative of a particular personality type. For example, thick lips are thought to suggest sensuality, whereas thin lips characterise meanness. The face is very much about who we are as a person.

It is the face that tells us how much two people like or are attracted to each other. Smiling, for example, is a very potent signal of positive feelings, although Ekman and Friesen (1982) distinguish between smiles that are felt, and those that are false or put on for the occasion. They found that false smiles do not involve the cheeks and eyes. During conversation smiles act as a reinforcer, encouraging the speaker to continue with a topic.

The face is also very important in expressing how we feel. Ekman (1982) identified seven main facial expressions of emotion. These are happiness, sadness, surprise, fear, anger, disgust and interest, which are shown by various movements of the cheeks, mouth, nose and brow. The mouth, because of its role in speech, is the most mobile part of the face. Other expressions include shame (Izard 1977), interest, startle (Ekman 1985) and puzzlement.

When these facial expressions are used by listeners they provide the speaker with feedback. It shows not only whether the listener is interested, surprised or disgusted by what they hear, but whether they have understood. The speaker is able to monitor these reactions, and adapt their communication accordingly.

The role of facial expression in signalling attitude and emotion means that it is a significant factor in the formation of relationships. This starts in babies with their first cry. This primitive response rapidly develops into a complex repertoire that allows the infant to signal a range of emotions by the age of six months (Izard 1978). The parent responds to these signals, and the child soon learns he can control his environment.

Perception of facial expression in others is also crucial to the child's social development. As early as three weeks, the baby starts to show an interest in his mother's face during feeding (Sheridan 1975). He shows recognition of family members by twenty months, and is able to point to their faces in a photograph by two years (Sheridan 1975).

Facial expressions are usually a response to an external stimulus, although a person may deliberately use them as a signal – for example, the teacher who uses a frown to show disapproval. This ability to make a pose with the face means that it is sometimes difficult to interpret a facial expression. People may attempt to hide their true feelings for a variety of reasons. The depressed host of a party may feel it is socially unacceptable to look sad, and therefore attempts to hide this by smiling. Other people are bound by cultural conventions that dictate how and when emotion is expressed. In Japan, for instance, negative emotions are usually hidden.

Sometimes people find it difficult to control their facial expression. The face may leak information about a person's true feelings. For instance, a person may look embarrassed when meeting someone with a disfiguring scar. Professionals working in a health care context need to monitor their facial expression carefully to prevent this type of leakage occurring.)

Facial expression, and in particular the facial features, also play a significant role in diagnosis. Abnormalities of the facial features are associated with a variety of congenital syndromes, for example the protruding tongue and open mouth associated with Down's syndrome (Northern and Downs 1974). Certain acquired neurological disorders affect facial expression. For instance, in Parkinson's disease the person develops a typical mask like expression, characterised by limited mobility that even affects smiling (Darly *et al.* 1975). Facial expression often indicates a disturbance of affect as in depressive illnesses (Gilroy and Holliday 1982). The face also shows a response to physiological states like pain, fatigue or cold.

Gesture

Argyle (1988) has defined gestures as those bodily movements intended as a form of communication. These include movements of the head, hands and other parts of the body. They are distinguishable from posture (Lamb and Watson 1979), which involves the whole of the body. As well as these intentional gestures there are movements that occur as an involuntary response to an object, other people or a specific event. For example, a person reacting to a shock might place their hand across the mouth. Morris (1978) described voluntary movements as primary gestures, and involuntary movements as secondary gestures.

Primary gestures are voluntary movements that a person uses with the intent of communicating a message to another person. There are three main primary gesture types:

1. **Emblems** (Ekman and Friesen 1969). These are gestures that have a direct verbal equivalent. For example, a wave of the hand during a parting means goodbye. Emblems tend to develop in situations where using speech would be impossible. Workers in the old cotton mills of northern England developed gestural systems of communication, because it was impossible to hear speech in the noisy machine rooms. Modern day equivalents are the systems used by the tic-tac men at the race track, airport controllers on the runway, and the police officer directing traffic. Although some of these gestural systems are elaborate, they are not to be confused with sign languages, which have a distinct grammar and vocabulary. (See more information on this in 'Working With Interpreters'.)

2. **Illustrators** (Ekman and Friesen 1969). These gestures are closely linked with speech, and serve to emphasise, clarify or add to the verbal content of the message. Illustrators are mainly made by movements of the hand. Argyle (1988) describes several different types of illustrator:

>   **Batons** – these movements emphasise the rhythm of speech. Bull and Connelly (1985) found that most points of stress in a sentence were accompanied by a movement of the head, hand or other part of the body. For example, a politician may stress key words in his speech by making a chopping movement with his hand.

>   **Pointing** – is a common gesture that infants as young as eighteen months are able to use (Murphy and Messer 1977). It is used to direct attention to either self or people, objects and events that are external.

>   **Spatial movements or relationships** – These gestures show either the movement or the position of objects and people. So a downward movement of the hands might accompany the sentence 'the balloon dropped like a stone.'

>   **Pictographs** – These gestures are used to show the shape of objects – a circular motion for a ball, a square for a box and so on.

>   **Ideographs** – These gestures are used to illustrate a line of thought.

>   **Bodily actions** – Gestures that are mimes of actual actions, for example – pretending to hit a ball with a cricket bat.

3. **Reinforcers.** These are gestures that help regulate the flow of conversation. For example, a nod of the head encourages the speaker to continue.

Secondary or incidental gestures (Morris 1978) are also important in communication even though they are not intentional. Gestures such as grooming the hair, fiddling or wringing the hands are all examples of involuntary gestures. Although they are not intended to communicate, Morris warns that they often send messages. This is termed 'leakage' – when our true feelings or attitudes are revealed despite what our overt signals are saying. So a young person may say 'I'm not worried about taking my driving test' whilst continually opening and closing his hands.

One group of involuntary gestures of particular significance to the health professional are those described as 'self-touching' actions (Freedman and Hoffman 1967). Examples include touching the face, scratching or gripping the hands together. These occur when people are experiencing intense emotions such as depression, elation or extreme anxiety, and are characterised by their lack of purpose (Trower *et al.* 1978). Interpreting these involuntary gestures is not a precise science, and care needs to be taken before attaching too much significance to these behaviours unless there is other supporting evidence.

Body posture

Posture refers to the position of the body and limbs (Wilkinson and Canter 1982), in particular, placement of the head, arms and legs, and the amount that the body leans forwards, backwards or sideways (Argyle 1988). There are endless combinations.

Many postures that individuals adopt are determined by the society in which they live (Lamb and Watson 1979). Social conventions dictate which positions are acceptable in different situations. Lying on the floor in an exercise class is regarded as normal behaviour, whereas lying on the floor in the office is usually frowned upon. Other postures are associated with particular ceremonies and special events. For example, a person might kneel in front of the monarch when they are knighted. Some postures occur more frequently in one culture than another; bowing for instance, is one behaviour used regularly in Japan but rarely in Britain. Each person will also develop a characteristic stance. This is influenced by personality, physical characteristics, health and even the type of footwear worn by the person.

Posture is of interest to health professionals as it signals the strength of a person's emotional response. This is expressed partly by the position of the body but also by its muscular tone. Depression is characterised by low tonus, and drooping head and shoulders (Trower *et al.* 1978), which gives an appearance of sadness and fatigue (Ingram *et al.* 1981). Mania and anxiety are associated with increased muscular tone. The body being held in an excessively stiff and upright manner.

Muscular tone is also significant in signalling different attitudes. The most dominant person in an interaction is likely to display a relaxed posture. If the subordinates were to take on an excessively relaxed posture, this would be interpreted as disrespect. This type of behaviour typifies some teenage reactions to authority figures such as teachers or police.

Mehrabian (1972) identified the following components of relaxation: asymmetrical positioning of the arms and legs, leaning back or to the side, and relaxed muscular tone. In contrast men will adopt a highly tense posture when threatened. This is characterised by a drawing up to their full height and expansion of the chest area.

Another dimension of posture is the open versus closed body positions. An open body position is seen as more friendly, warm and inviting. The person usually sits or stands closer to the other person, with arms and legs open rather than folded or crossed. They face the other person, leaning forwards slightly. A closed body position is just the opposite. Arms and legs are crossed as if to protect the body from attack. The person leans back and might attempt to distance themselves. If this is not possible they will turn their body away. A closed position is usually interpreted as less friendly and even rejecting.

During conversation the listener's posture is another form of feedback for the speaker. Interest is conveyed by leaning forward with legs drawn back; whereas boredom is associated with a lowered head, leaning back and outstretched legs (Bull 1987). Body cues are also important in bringing about the end of the conversation. Feet and legs are pointed at the door (Knapp et al. 1973), and weight is shifted from one foot to the other (Bull 1983).

Head movements

This section will consider the significance of the position, orientation and movement of the head during social interaction. They may seem insignificant but they serve several important roles. Argyle (1978) has described head movements as a special type of gesture. Like other gestures, head movements need to be considered in context (Lamb and Watson 1979) to determine their meaning.

During conversation the listener shows that they are attending by offering encouragement through occasional single or double nods. Research has shown that these head nods act as reinforcers, which encourage the speaker to continue talking or talk more about a particular topic (Krasner 1958). Head movements also regulate turntaking during conversation. By rapidly nodding their head (Argyle 1978) or turning their head away (Duncan and Fiske 1977), the listener signals to the speaker that they want to have a turn at talking.

These same movements of the head are used by speakers to accompany their speech. In English a yes response is accompanied by a nod of the head, whereas a shake of the head indicates disagreement or refusal. It is interesting to note that these movements are not universal. In Greece a toss of the head usually accompanies a negative response. Like other gestures these two movements of the head can be used to replace speech. For instance when we recognise a friend or neighbour on the other side of the street, we might nod our head as a form of greeting.

Head movements are closely linked with posture. The position of the head, like overall posture, provides clues about how a person is feeling. For instance, a lowered head with a slumped posture might indicate depression (Waxer 1974).

The orientation of the head is also meaningful. People turn their heads towards something that interests them (Izard 1977), often leaning forward with the whole body (Bull 1987). A listener who is bored may lower or turn their head away, sit with their head tilted to one side or even resting on their hand (Bull 1987).

It is also an indicator of the relative importance of individuals. When a person talks to someone of higher status, the head tends to be raised up. In a study by Spiegel and Machotka (1974) head orientation was more significant than body orientation in signalling dominance.

2

Paralinguistic Features of Communication

Quality of voice

Each of us has a characteristic way of speaking. Our friends and family would probably be able to identify us by voice alone. Voice quality is one of the dimensions that provides us with this unique vocal identity. Resonance is one feature of voice that affects its quality. Some voices can be described as rich and full, whereas others seem thin and reedy. Apart from being more pleasant to the ear, a resonating voice projects farther.

Voice quality may be disrupted in some cases. A breathy voice occurs when air escapes during phonation. It was a characteristic of many fifty's film stars, including Marilyn Monroe. This type of voice quality is perceived as sexy or feminine. However, it is not an efficient way of producing voice. In most cases poor voice quality like a harsh, tense or hoarse voice, is unpleasant for the listener. People experiencing a change in voice quality need to seek medical advice.

Volume

Speakers need to maintain an adequate level of volume in order to be heard and understood. Despite this, individuals show a wide variation in this vocal characteristic. Hence descriptions of a 'soft delivery' or 'bellowing voice'. The speaker also has to adjust their volume to suit different situations. So a quiet voice is used in a library or a church, whereas shouting is more appropriate for a football match.

Public speakers use sudden increases in loudness to maintain the audience's attention or add emphasis to their message. Speeches by politicians illustrate this technique very effectively!

A change in volume may also be an expression of how the person is feeling; different emotions are characterised by changes in volume – for instance, a loud voice is associated with anger, and a quiet voice with sadness. Volume also signals information about our attitudes – a dominant person is more likely to use a louder voice. Volume is linked closely with pitch and rate of speech (Scherer 1981). So a high pitch and fast rate of speech are associated with anger.

Intonation and pitch

The pitch of the voice provides the listener with a clue to the speaker's age and gender. A male speaker usually has a low pitched voice compared with the characteristically high pitch of the female speaker. Children have a high pitch; which decreases with age in both males and females (Siegman 1987). The deepening or 'breaking' of the male voice during puberty is particularly noticeable.

Each speaker will use a range of frequencies during normal speech. This is known as their pitch range. Changes in the level and range of pitch convey information about the feelings and attitudes of the speaker. For example, it tends to be raised with a more variable and wider pitch range when a person has lost their temper (Scherer 1986). A low pitch is associated with dominance, and submissiveness with a high pitch (Frick 1985).

The most significant role of pitch is its ability to alter meaning. During speech a person will use a range of pitch levels, the movement between these levels being called falls and rises. These movements form a pattern called intonation. In English, these patterns have two main functions: to emphasise key words for the listener and to distinguish between different types of sentence (Gimson 1980). Look at how the meaning changes when the emphasis is moved between words in the following phrase – 'My cats are in the bedroom?'. (Note the symbol + denotes which word is stressed.)

'Are your dogs in the bedroom?' –

'No. My +cats are in the bedroom' (Not my dogs.)

'Are your cats in the kitchen?' –

'No. My cats are in the +bedroom' (Not the kitchen.)

'Are Dawn's cats in the bedroom?'

'No. +My cats are in the bedroom' (Not Dawn's cats.)

Intonation also helps the listener to differentiate between various types of sentence. For example, a statement like 'The library is closed' changes into a question if the word 'closed' is spoken with a rising intonation, although it cannot be assumed that every question has a rising pitch.

People learn to recognise the meanings of different intonational patterns; however, their interpretations are not always reliable. This is due to the influence of context and speaker characteristics on the meaning of intonation.

Rate of speech

The rate of speech is a determining factor in the clarity of a speaker. We all know that we can say a tongue twister without making a mistake, if we slow down and articulate carefully. Once we speed up it is very difficult to prevent any errors. Besides losing precision we also disrupt the natural rhythm of the sentence. Both these things make it very difficult for the listener to understand. This is an exaggerated way of showing what happens when we talk too fast.

The reverse of this problem is the speaker who talks too slowly. This creates problems as the listener is able to process speech much faster than the speaker can produce it (Armstrong 1984). Normally this gap between production and processing allows the listener to assimilate and process information. If the gap is too long they are likely to lose interest and find it difficult to maintain concentration. The natural rhythm may also be distorted.

The rate of speech, like other vocal features, expresses different emotions and attitudes. When someone loses their temper, their rate of speech will be faster. Sadness is associated with a slowing down of speech. Dominance is also signalled by a slower rate.

Tone of voice

What we perceive as tone is really a combination of different vocal aspects that include pitch, volume, rate, voice quality and rhythm. Each of these features can be varied to create different combinations. These are used to express emotion and convey information about attitudes. Argyle (1988) describes a friendly tone as 'high pitched, with a lot of gentle upward pitch variation, pure tones, and regular rhythm' (p.146).

Sometimes the tone of our voice suggests a different message from the words we are using. This is known as a mixed message. The listener has to decide which one to believe. Usually it is the paralinguistic information that is accepted as revealing the real intention of the speaker. This is because it is much harder to control our voices, and our true feelings 'leak' out. It is important for health professionals to be aware of this, and to monitor their communication when dealing with clients.

Conversational oil

Conversational oil refers to words, phrases and vocalisations like 'mm-hmm', 'that's right' and 'I see'. They are the vocal equivalent of head nodding during conversation; telling the speaker that she has been heard and understood. Depending on the choice of words they may also indicate the degree of interest by the listener, and whether they are in agreement with the speaker. Like other social reinforcers, it is important they are used appropriately. Think about the interviews you have attended. Did any of the interviewers respond with a series of 'mmm's? Did you feel you were being taken seriously? Too many automatic responses dilute the effect of this type of feedback. The use of other non-verbal signals along with these phrases is important. For example, a smile with 'that's right', or a head nod with 'mm-hmm'. Used appropriately these reinforcers encourage the speaker to continue and expand on their topic. Hence the term 'conversational oil', which refers to their ability to maintain the flow of the conversation.

3

Verbal Communication

What makes a good verbal communicator?

Verbal communication refers to the words and phrases of spoken language. Its complex and multidimensional nature means that any description needs to be approached from a number of different perspectives. The main parameters of language are content, structure, form and use of language:

Content

This relates to the meaning of verbal language. It may also be referred to as the topic or message; and in linguistics it is known as semantics.

There are different types of meaning. Look at these well-known expressions:

> 'Too many cooks spoil the broth'

> 'A stitch in time saves nine'

> 'Every cloud has a silver lining'

We are all familiar with the underlying message in these idioms. This type of meaning is known as idiomatic.

Metaphors are another way of expressing meaning by using terms that do not directly apply to the subject. 'You are the jewel in my crown' is one example where the meaning is inferred.

Most of the time we take the literal meaning of words, although this will vary between contexts. The request 'Can you open the door?' when used to a child may mean 'have you got the strength' or 'can you reach the handle', whereas a similar request from one lift passenger to another may mean 'I am stuck here at the back of this crowded lift, can you press the button and let me out'. So context is also important in determining the meaning of a sentence.

Misunderstandings arise when words are taken out of context, or a literal meaning is applied to an idiom or metaphor. A lecturer, who did not speak

English as a first language, was baffled by the secretary's comments that 'The students are a bit thin on the ground, today'.

Structure of the language

This refers to the way in which words are put together to form sentences. Each language has its own rules that govern which words can occur together and in what order. This is known as the syntax or grammar of a language. Moving, adding or omitting words will change the meaning of a sentence.

The structure of a sentence sometimes results in ambiguity. For example, 'the traffic warden stopped the car at the junction'. Was the traffic warden driving the car? Or did she stop a car being driven by somebody else? Sometimes the use of a particular word creates the possibility of more than one interpretation. The subject matter of this lecture is unclear: 'the nurses received a talk on sterilisation'. Is the topic sterilisation of instruments or sterilisation as a form of birth control?

Word structure

This is about the structure of individual words. For example, the single noun 'boy' is made into a plural by adding an 's', and the ending 'ed' is added to the verb 'walk' when it is used to denote the past tense. Like the sentence, word structure is rule based.

Form of the language

This refers to the way in which sounds are combined to make words. Sounds are used contrastively, so that a change in one sound alters the meaning and function of a word. For example, by swapping the vowel sound in 'cat' with a series of different vowel sounds, we get numerous other words that include 'cut' 'cot' 'cart' and 'curt'. Sometimes this will alter the grammatical class of the word. 'Cat' is a noun (name), whereas the word 'cut' can be used as a noun or a verb (doing word).

In written English the spoken word is represented by letters. Sometimes people confuse the sounds of speech with the names of these letters. However, there is a difference. Compare the sound of [p], with the letter p (pronounced as 'pea').

Sometimes one sound is represented in ordinary spelling as two letters. So the sound at the beginning of shop 'sh' (like the sound used to hush somebody) is represented by 's' and 'h'. Some sounds have several different written spellings. The vowel sound in the word pea is the same vowel sound found in <u>see</u>, <u>piece</u> and <u>key</u>.

To avoid confusion sounds have their own symbols, which are used when speech is transcribed. These are known as phonetic symbols. The symbol for 'sh' is [∫], and the vowel sound 'ee' is represented by [i].

Use of language

The verbal elements of a language are used in many different ways. In a similar way to non-verbal and paralinguistic features they:

- give information
- seek information
- express feelings
- convey information about attitudes
- establish and maintain relationships
- regulate social interaction.

Besides these functions, verbal language also enables us:

- To direct the actions of others
- To express ideas
- To form concepts
- To develop logical arguments
- To describe objects, people, events and feelings
- To solve problems
- To talk about objects and people not present
- To talk about events in the past or the future
- To debate and discuss issues
- To hypothesise
- To create make-believe
- To develop novel ideas
- To make threats
- To give promises.

And numerous other examples.

Style or register

The vocabulary, form and structure of language used by individuals varies between different social contexts. The main difference is between formal and informal settings. This is clearly illustrated by comparing the street talk of children in the school playground with the formal vocabulary and language used by the same children when addressing their headteacher. Recognising these differences and being able to adapt accordingly are part of successful communication.

What are those special qualities that make a person excel in their verbal communication? I asked some of my friends and colleagues – 'What makes a good verbal communicator?' Here are some of their thoughts and mine:

✧ A clear message

'relevant' 'having something to communicate to others' 'clear message' 'interesting'

Part of the skill in verbal communication is being able to organise your thoughts and present them in a logical way. Irrelevant details need to be omitted and essential ideas highlighted. You also need to know the interests of your listener before you can make your message relevant.

✧ Talking to the person, and not at them

'looks you straight in the eye' 'makes contact' 'feel you are being spoken to'

Eye-contact was stressed by everybody as very important. One person said that they would quickly dismiss any message from someone who avoided looking at them.

✧ A good listener

'making space for them to reply' 'taking turns' 'listening and responding' 'not interrupting'

This is an essential skill, and just as important as any of the verbal elements. The coherence of a conversation relies on a shared topic, which the participants are able to maintain through several speaking turns. It is necessary for each person to listen before they are able to respond appropriately. When this interchange breaks down the conversation becomes disjointed and frustrating. Examples will come easily to mind.

✧ Understanding the needs of the listener

'appropriate vocabulary and language' 'not being talked down to' 'spoken to at your level'

Vocabulary and language have to be adapted according to the needs of the listener as well as the context.

This applies to the complexity of language as well to the amount of information.

✧ Appreciation of the listener

'feeling your opinions matter' 'genuinely interested in audience' 'showing they enjoy talking to the other person' 'giving time for each person' 'not being egocentric'

The person who shows appreciation of the listener, is more likely to gain and hold their attention, be perceived positively, and elicit longer and in depth contributions.

✧ Personal characteristics

'pleasant' 'enthusiastic' 'non-threatening' 'consistent in their views' 'vital'

The personal qualities of an individual influence our perception of them as a speaker. Two people may have very different views of the same speaker, one thinking them directive and rigid, while the other finds them logical and organised. Sometimes it is impossible to define these qualities exactly. However, there do seem to be some common characteristics, which are described above.

✧ Getting feedback

'gets feedback on effectiveness of message' 'checking with the audience'

The speaker needs to check constantly on the effectiveness of their communication. Looking at body language and listening to responses will provide feedback. A more active approach is to ask questions to check the message has been understood.

✧ Vocal qualities

'not loud, or hectoring' 'not a droning voice' 'not shrill' 'clear voice' 'speaks up'

The overall consensus was the need for a pleasant, interesting and lively voice.

Think of people you admire as speakers. What are the qualities that attract you to them? Sometimes people are good in one situation, and not in another. Is that the case with anyone you know?

Advanced verbal skills relevant to professionals

A prerequisite for selection to any training course in the health care professions is good interpersonal skills. Mature entrants also bring the benefit of a variety of life experiences. This often leads students to wonder why communication skills are included on the curriculum. The answer is that the health professional needs to develop advanced social skills. These are required by the nature of the work, which places special demands on the individual. She has to learn new ways of coping in a variety of situations. Here are some thought provokers:

✧ *Health professionals meet many different people during the course of their work*

Write down all the people you have contact with during the course of the day. Students can try this during a practical placement. You will be surprised by the range of people.

✧ *Health professionals are involved in a variety of difficult situations*
These include:
- bereavement
- chronic illness
- diagnosis of disability
- progressive disease
- surgery
- mental illness.

What difficult situations form part of your working life? How often do you have to deal with these?

✧ *Look at this list of the skills required in providing health care:*
- Providing information
- Offering emotional support
- Instructing or teaching the client
- Relieving anxiety and stress
- Helping the client to express their needs, concerns and desires
- Providing reassurance
- Controlling behaviour (i.e. aggressive, unsocial)

- ○ Dealing with the client's embarrassment
- ○ Imparting bad news.

How many more can you think of?

✧ *The client forms a unique part of any interaction. The person's physical, emotional or psychological needs will interfere with their ability to assimilate, process and respond to information. The health professional learns to adapt their communication according to these needs.*

What are the needs of your clients? How do you adapt your communication to meet these needs?

✧ *The primary role of the health professional is a clinical one. However, there are numerous other roles that are required besides that of the clinician.*

What additional roles are you expected to carry out?

PART TWO

Interviews

4. Purpose of Interviews

5. Scene Setting

6. Gathering Information

7. Involving the Interviewee

8. Completing the Interview

9. Dealing with Difficult Situations

10. Working with Interpreters

11. Interviewing Skills in Context:
    11.1. *Clinical Interviews*
    11.2. *Appraisal Interviews*
    11.3. *Recruitment Interviews*
    11.4. *Grievance and Disciplinary Interviews*
    11.5. *Interviews with the Media*

Interviewing

Every health professional is required to develop expertise in interviewing clients to obtain clinical data, offer advice and discuss treatment. Through the interviewing process they are also able to establish and maintain a relationship with the client. These clinical interviews form the focus of the communication training for students studying health care.

However, the clinical interview is only one example of the many situations that require interviewing skills. The health professional is involved in a variety of interviews during their working life. Sometimes they will act as interviewer, at other times they will be interviewed. Some examples of interview situations for health professionals are:

- Taking a *case history* from a client
- Attending an *appraisal* interview with their line manager
- Chairing a *selection* panel for a new post
- Responding to questions from a local *journalist*
- Interviewing a member of staff as part of a *disciplinary hearing*.

Selection interviews are a common experience. These act like gateways through which the individual must pass, first to obtain entrance into employment, and then to make progress within their career. The significance of these interviews makes it imperative that individuals learn to maximise their skills.

Career progression will bring the clinician extra responsibilities. This may entail recruiting staff, acting as an appraiser and possibly participating in grievance or disciplinary interviews. The ability to perform well in these situations is crucial to the organisation as a whole, as well as to the staff group and the clients.

Traditionally there has been less emphasis on offering training for non-clinical interviews. This is slowly starting to change with the introduction of in-service training for professional skills.

The main part of this section looks at common skills and processes that relate to these different types of interview. It includes the following topics:

Purpose of interviews

The different types of interview. The special nature of the interview.

Scene setting

How to set the scene for your interview. Making the best of your environment. Setting time boundaries. Negotiating an agenda. Checklist for preparing an interview.

Gathering information

How to collect information. Tips on effective listening. Giving the interview a structure. Encouraging the interviewee. Maintaining control over the interview.

Involving the interviewee

Barriers to effective information giving. Using appropriate language. How to structure your information giving. Making sure your message has been understood.

Completing the interview

Skills of summarising. Planning future action. Clarifying understanding.

Dealing with difficult situations

How to develop the skills required to deal with difficult situations that arise during interviews.

Working with interpreters

Why you need professional interpretation. Communication in the interpreted interview. Guidelines for working with an interpreter. Interpreters for the sensory impaired. Checklist for booking an interpreter.

The final part of this section looks at interviews in context. Use this section for advice on specific situations:

Clinical interviews

How to elicit accurate and full information. Effective information giving. Guidelines for adult and paediatric case histories. Dealing with difficult clients.

Appraisal interviews

Making the right preparation. The roles of the appraiser and the appraisee. Improving communication within appraisal systems.

Grievance and disciplinary interview

Special characteristics of these types of interview. Organising the interview. Strategies for maximising communication.

Recruitment interviews

RECRUITING A CANDIDATE

Writing job descriptions and specifications. Advice on developing a job information pack. Interviewing the candidate.

APPLYING FOR A POST

Writing a curriculum vitae. Tips on completing an application form. Dressing for the interview. Communication in the interview. Checklist for recruitment interviews.

Interviews with the media

Preparing for your interview. How to communicate with the media. Thinking about your image.

4

Purpose of Interviews

An interview is a structured verbal exchange between two or more people, the purpose of which will vary according to the context. It is possible to identify some common aims that are applicable to all interviews. These are:

- establishing and maintaining a relationship
- gathering information
- conveying information
- offering support.

In a clinical setting, interviews are also part of the diagnostic process, and in some instances a therapy medium in themselves.

The purpose of the interview will determine the content. This may range from a discussion of factual information or goal setting to more subjective areas such as attitudes and feelings.

Interviews have a formalised structure. The time, venue and duration are agreed in advance; and the interview is conducted according to a recognised set of procedures. The exact format of the meeting will depend on the context. Generally an interview is a meeting between two people – the interviewer and the interviewee. Occasionally there are additional participants. A selection interview may have a panel of interviewers; and a clinical interview may involve the family or significant others, not just the client.

Interviews are distinguished from ordinary conversations by the fact that most of the flow of information is in one direction. So, a candidate in a selection interview may be asked about his hobbies, but is usually restricted from asking about the interests of the panel. This flow of information is usually directed by one person – the interviewer. But this is not an absolute rule. A good appraisal interview will encourage an exchange of ideas and information.

The content of an interview will vary according to the context and the purpose of the meeting. In an appraisal the discussion will centre on work performance, goals and objectives. The content of a clinical interview may focus on the feelings and attitudes of the client.

Summary Points

- An interview is a structured verbal exchange whose main purpose is information gathering.

- Depending on the context the interview may also serve to establish and maintain relationships, convey information and offer support.

- The organisation and structure of an interview are usually agreed in advance.

- The content of an interview will vary according to the context and the purpose of the meeting.

5

Scene Setting

The design of the set often makes the difference between the success or failure of a theatre production. Space, lighting and colour are used to create the right atmosphere. Props are positioned carefully to assist and enhance the performance of the actors. The scene is set. Like the stage manager you need to set the scene for your interview.

Environment

First impressions are important. Careful consideration needs to be given to where the interview takes place, as well as the way in which it begins. This includes the reception and waiting areas as well as the interview room. Who will greet people? Is there a waiting area? How comfortable is it? Make sure the interview room is clearly sign posted. Place your name, title and details of the interview on the door. This helps to orientate the interviewee, and it also informs other staff that the room is occupied.

Setting up the interview room

Think about where your interview will take place. It may be a hospital clinic room; a school medical room; an office or a board room. A clinical setting is associated with illness. A medical room is reminiscent of childhood vaccinations. An office or a board room has an air of formality; the atmosphere is one of business rather than health care. What images do these rooms conjure up for you? People will vary in their responses to the same setting, depending on their previous experience and their reason for being there. As an interviewer you need to be aware of these reactions.

Your choice of accommodation is influenced by the purpose of your interview, the limitations of your working environment and personal preference. Even when you have little choice over where you conduct your interviews, there are ways of adapting the setting to make it more conducive to your needs.

Think about what impression you want the interviewee to make of you, your profession and your organisation. Remove any clutter that might distract the interviewee. At the very least your desk must be clear. Are you giving positive or negative messages? Check for out of date material on the walls or notice boards.

As health professionals we sometimes have to work in temporary or shared accommodation. For instance, the room for your selection interviews may have large pieces of technical equipment. Dual purpose rooms pose a challenge. How can you alter the atmosphere using only temporary measures? Screens can transform any room. Use them to hide any extraneous furniture, equipment or even sinks. If you are working in a large room, like an unused hospital ward, you need to make the space smaller. Group chairs in a circle using a corner to give a cosy feeling. Screen unused areas with rows of large, leafy plants if you plan to be there for some time.

The type of furniture and how it is positioned will signal to the interviewee information about how the interview is likely to be conducted. Avoid extremes of height or comfort when choosing seating, or having any other obvious disparity between yourself and the interviewee. Arrange the lay-out of the room to suit your purpose. Position chairs away from any windows so that people are not distracted by movement outside or blinded by sunlight.

Preparation

The amount and type of preparation required will depend on the nature of your interview and your previous experience. Make sure you are familiar with the relevant procedures. In some interviews, the participants are expected to adhere to a formalised set of procedures. Grievance and disciplinary hearings are two examples of situations where failure to comply with the regulations may call into question the whole proceedings. Other interviews require careful thought about the process of gathering information. So, in a clinical situation, the interviewer will need to elicit a detailed case history. For an appraisal the interviewer needs to gather information before the actual appraisal interview. Whatever the type of interview, make sure you have an outline plan of what you intend to achieve.

Time boundaries

Timing is a very important aspect of interviews. It includes the scheduled start of the interview; the expected duration; and the punctuality of the participants in both starting and ending the interview. You need to aim for a mutually agreed starting time whenever possible. This increases the chance of your interviewee attending on time. Try to anticipate their needs. A candidate for a job interview may want an afternoon appointment if they have to travel from another part of the country. A young mother may prefer a morning dental appointment while her children are at nursery. It is not always possible to make an educated guess at suitable appointment times. In one of my clinics a mother refused a Tuesday morning appointment, saying that was the day she did her washing. I was at first puzzled why the washing needed to be done on this particularly day. I later found out she lived in a block of flats where tenants were allocated the use of the laundry only on certain days. The moral of the tale is always to confirm the convenience of appointments with the interviewee.

You also need to make the expected duration of the interview clear. This helps people organise their commitments around the interview slot. If a client or job applicant is worrying about picking up children from school they will not be participating fully in the interview. It also allows the interviewee to decide how to use the available time. If they know the interview will shortly end, they can prioritise what they are going to say. For instance, they might have a specific query. Mutual responsibility for using the time is particularly relevant to counselling sessions. In this situation there is a danger of the client becoming over reliant on the therapist making all the decisions. When the client knows the session length they can exercise some control over what happens.

Punctuality is a thorny issue in the health service. Managers are constantly seeking to improve waiting times. Statistics are regularly collected. At the same time there is pressure to increase the number of appointments. It is frustrating to be kept waiting, as anyone who has attended a hospital out-patients department will know. How would you rate yourself on time-keeping? Do your interviews always start and finish on time? The nature of health care means that unexpected problems arise that interfere with sched-ules. Sometimes it is a question of trying to please everyone at the same time. There is a sense of an unwritten obligation to answer the phone at any time, or see visitors and colleagues who have no appointment.

Reducing interruptions will improve the timing of your interviews. Try these tips:

- ○ Make it clear to colleagues and clients the times that you are available.
- ○ Warn the switch board that you will not be receiving calls while you are interviewing; or use an answering machine to take your messages.
- ○ Enlist the help of your receptionist or secretary to keep unexpected visitors at bay.
- ○ Provide the receptionist with a list of your appointments, so they can deal with cancellations or enquiries.
- ○ Finally place a large sign with 'Please Do Not Disturb' on the door!

Other people will learn to respect your time boundaries if you are consistent about using them. This is not only good time management, but essential if your interviews are to be satisfactory for the interviewee.

Introductions

At the beginning of a social encounter participants engage in some form of greeting. Any spoken remarks are usually accompanied by non-verbal behaviours such as smiling, shaking hands, and mutual eye-contact. In an interview, where one person is being invited into the territory of another, comments specifically intended to welcome the interviewee are also used. These are usually followed by a few non-specific comments regarding the weather or travel, which are intended to put the interviewee at ease.

If you fail to use these opening moves, you will appear rude or brusque. Failure to establish rapport at this stage of the interview can adversely affect communication and hinder a successful outcome.

Apart from initiating interactions, introductions also serve a number of other specific purposes. As an interviewer you will want to:

- ○ Establish a rapport with the interviewee
- ○ Introduce yourself and explain your role
- ○ Find out what expectations the interviewee has about your role
- ○ Find out what expectations the interviewee has about the content of the interview
- ○ Seek agreement on the purpose and nature of the interview
- ○ Reinforce links with previous interviews (if appropriate).

If the interview is a follow-up to a previous meeting, a link needs to be made with what has happened before. The previous discussion can be briefly reviewed. One or two statements about what was discussed will suffice. For example, 'Last time we met we discussed the various treatment options. As you will remember they were – surgery, drugs or radiotherapy. We now have the test results that we need to help us make a decision.'

If you have not met the interviewee before you will need to introduce yourself and explain your role. This is particularly important in clinical interviews, where the client may have very little information available to them about the interview. Describe your role using terms that the interviewee will understand. One person thought that the 'registrar' admitting her to hospital was the person who recorded people's names. They were not familiar with the job titles used by doctors. What is your job title? Would everyone know what it means? Think about the sorts of information represented by your title and grade. How can this information be explained in everyday language?

By defining your role you demonstrate to the interviewee that you have the necessary expertise. It is also an opportunity for identifying any misconceptions the interviewee may have about what you are offering. Misunderstandings of this sort can cause anger or embarrassment for the interviewee if they later become aware of any error. Until there is a mutual understanding of the role of the interviewer communication will be less than satisfactory.

Every interview has an agenda. In some interviews this agenda will be flexible and negotiated between the participants. Other interviews require a formal structure, and the purpose and nature of the interview are determined in advance. Occasionally there is a 'hidden' agenda. This happens when one or more people have specific goals that they have not made explicit. For example, the employee who attends an appraisal interview with the single purpose of complaining about a colleague. Even in a formal situation where the agenda is fixed, there still needs to be a general agreement as to the purpose of the interview. Otherwise there is no point in continuing with the interview. By expressing your intentions and asking the interviewee about their expectations you initiate the process of agenda setting. Part of this process is explaining the rules. The interviewee needs to know what will happen and the sequence in which it will occur; for example, basic things such as when to ask questions, to more serious issues of confidentiality. Once you have established an agenda you can start the main business of your meeting.

Summary Points

- First impressions are important. They influence the expectations of the participants and the subsequent interaction.

- The environment in which the interview takes place will affect the quality of your communication. Reception and the waiting area are just as important as the interview room.

- Arrange the interview room to maximise communication.

- Reduce distractions in the room and minimise interruptions.

- Familiarise yourself with the interview procedures. Plan a rough outline of your interview.

- Make sure that any necessary leaflets, forms or other materials are available in the interview room.

- Timing is a very important aspect of interviews. Arrange a mutually acceptable time with the interviewee, and make it clear how long the interview will last.

- Use greetings and general chat to establish rapport with the interviewee.

- Introduce yourself and explain your role in terms that will be understood by the interviewee.

- Make your intentions clear to the interviewee and establish their expectations of the interview.

- Communicate the purpose of the interview and the general aims of the session. Negotiate specific objectives if this is relevant.

Checklist for Scene Setting

Organising the Interview

- ☐ Have you agreed a date and time with the interviewee?
- ☐ Have you booked a suitable room?
- ☐ Is it arranged to your satisfaction?
- ☐ Is the interview room clearly signposted?
- ☐ Does the receptionist or secretary have a list of your appointments?
- ☐ Is there a clear procedure for greeting interviewees?
- ☐ Have you taken steps to reduce distractions and interruptions?
- ☐ Have you informed the switchboard to hold your calls or take messages?
- ☐ Are colleagues aware when and where you are interviewing?

Preparation

- ☐ Have you gathered together the relevant materials?
- ☐ Do you know the procedures relevant to this interview?
- ☐ Have you done all the necessary preparation?

Introductions

- ☐ Have you introduced yourself?
- ☐ Have you explained your role?
- ☐ Have you made the purpose of the interview clear?
- ☐ Have you established the expectations of the interviewee?
- ☐ Have you discussed the likely outcomes?

6

Gathering Information

One of the primary purposes of an interview is to gather information. This is achieved by a number of different methods. Some of these are used before the interview, whereas others are integral to the interviewing process itself.

The following is a list of the methods commonly used to gather information before the interview:

- questionnaires
- forms
- historical information
- specific recommendations
- information from other agencies.

Questionnaires

Many people favour the use of a questionnaire to gain specific information before the interview. A range of question styles can be used to elicit information.

Yes or no response

These questions are designed to elicit either a positive or negative response. They are worded in such a way as to avoid ambiguity or the necessity for the answer to be qualified in any way. Examples would be 'Do you suffer from indigestion?' 'Do you have any bleeding from the ears?' 'Have you got a current driving licence?' By structuring the questions in this way, the interviewer is able to elicit information about a predetermined set of items.

Wh- type questions

These are questions that require a specific one or two word response. Examples would include 'When did you have your operation?' 'What contraceptive are you using?' 'Where did you train?' The questioner still has a lot of control over what information is elicited, although there is more variety in the response. Wh questions are a useful alternative, when it would be impracticable to use a yes/no one. An example is 'Where did you train?', which would require numerous 'Did you train at...?' questions.

Multiple-choice

These are questions that supply a choice of answer. They may be in the form of a forced alternative like 'Do you wear a behind-the-ear or a body worn hearing aid?' The interviewee merely has to select which is the correct response. Sometimes a choice of responses are supplied. So a question might be worded as 'Do you use a barrier/oral/rhythm method of contraception?'.

Forms

These might have questions worded in a similar fashion to the questionnaire, but they also designed so that specific information can be listed. There might be a space for qualifications or for details of employment history.

Application forms are traditionally used in recruiting. They provide a way of gathering standard information that can be used to make comparisons between candidates.

Forms are also used in other types of interviews, particularly appraisals. The appraisee being asked to list his duties and responsibilities. In this case it is also a way of guiding the appraisee in their preparation, and stimulating thought about their work performance.

Historical information

Sometimes an interviewer has access to information from previous interviews. An appraiser will have last year's appraisal records. A clinician will have a record of the client's previous medical history. If information of this nature is available it needs to be read. This will not only save time, but may also avoid embarrassing or distressing the interviewee. The question 'How many children do you have?' seems innocuous. However, if a child has died in the family, this question becomes a potential source of distress.

Specific recommendations

These may come in the form of a reference or a testimonial to good character. All recruitment procedures make use of references, one of which is usually the last employer or training establishment. In a disciplinary, character references may be produced as evidence. These sorts of recommendations provide information about the attitudes and personality of the interviewee, which may be difficult to evaluate in other ways.

Other agencies

A clinical interview is often assisted by information supplied by other agencies involved with the client. So a developmental assessment of a child is greatly aided by reports of the child's progress from therapists, health visitors and local medical officers. The referral letter itself is also a source of information.

Results of tests

The results of a test provide the interviewer with objective information on the performance or status of the interviewee. There are two main interviews where tests are used as a source of information.

In the clinical interview, tests are a familiar and routine part of clinical procedures. It is essential that the clinician has seen all the relevant results before the interview.

Tests are sometimes used in recruitment. They assess a range of qualities in the job applicant from knowledge and skills to attributes required by the post holder. So, a secretary might be asked to complete a typing or shorthand test. A salesperson may have to complete psychometric tests on personality. Testing of this sort is not a widespread practice in the health service.

Pros and cons of collecting information before the interview

There are obvious advantages to collecting information before the interview. Some information is a determining factor in whether an interview occurs or not. Information from a job applicant, for example, is used as part of the selection process for interview.

The benefits will depend on the type of information and the purpose of the interview. Here are some pros:

- The information provides a focus for the discussion.
- The interviewer is able to prepare more thoroughly.
- There is less possibility of any details being overlooked.
- It saves time.
- It stimulates the interviewee to prepare for the interview.
- It allows the interviewee a chance to set the agenda by stating their concerns.

Despite the advantages of gathering information before the interview, there are some drawbacks. Questionnaires and forms pose difficulties for people whose first language is not English or those who have a literacy problem. Providing written material in a range of languages that reflect the cultural mix of the area will help breakdown any language barrier.

The other major disadvantage is the effect of bias. We know that interviewers have a tendency to recruit job candidates with a similar background and experience – the mirror image syndrome. Information that reinforces this perception may well influence the outcome of the interview. This is also true for other interviews. For instance, referral information about a client may be biased (Thompson, Newell and Dryden 1991). Interviewers need to be aware that they will be influenced by the information they receive about the interviewee, and that the actual information itself may be biased.

Developing an appropriate format for questionnaires and forms is notoriously difficult. By definition they must have a standard format with a standard vocabulary. Not all the questions are likely to be appropriate to the respondent. And unlike the questions asked in the interview, there is no opportunity for language to be modified to meet the needs of the respondent. No matter how well the questions are worded there is always the possibility that they may be misunderstood. Therefore information gained in this way always needs to be verified during the interview.

Some questions may not be suitable for use on forms. Questions that are likely to arouse strong reactions or raise a query in the mind of the respondent are best asked during the interview. Then the interviewer can respond appropriately by answering questions and dealing with the fears and concerns of the interviewee.

One of the difficulties with written material is that it is not possible to monitor the response of the person to the questions. People also have more time to think about their reply, and are therefore more likely to write what they view as an acceptable answer.

Interview

The bulk of information gathering takes place during the interview. Various methods can be used by the interviewer to elicit information. These are by:

- Observation
- Asking questions
- Encouraging contributions from the interviewee.

Observation

The interview situation provides the interviewer with the opportunity of observing the interviewee. Observation is about both watching and listening.

Watching

Information about feelings, attitudes and reactions are expressed through various non-verbal behaviours. (These behaviours are discussed in detail in the first section of the book.) Here is a brief reminder of those aspects of body language that are important signals during interaction.

Posture

How does the person walk into the room? (Head down with shoulders slouched or an upright posture with head up and shoulders back.)

How do they sit? (Leaning forwards; leaning backwards; hunched over; relaxed; tense; in a closed or open position.)

Eye-contact

How much does the person look at you? When do they look at you? Is eye-gaze averted?

Facial expression

Does the person smile? How often? What do they smile about?

Are they frowning?

What expression do they have? (Interested; bored; sad; anxious.)

The purpose of your interview will determine the significance of what you observe. In a clinical interview, observation of the client's physical appearance is important. In an appraisal you will want to observe the appraisee's reactions to any proposals.

Effective listening skills

Privacy and a distraction free environment create the right atmosphere for effective listening both by yourself and the interviewee. You will be able to concentrate if interruptions are reduced, and the interviewee will also feel attention is focused on them. Reinforce this feeling by using appropriate listening behaviour. Looking at the person is a strong non-verbal signal of attentiveness; as are nods of the head, smiling and leaning forwards slightly. Using body language in this way will show that you are prepared to listen.

Watch the interviewee. Do they appear to be listening? Remember that people who look as if they are attending are not always listening. Do any of the following situations ring a bell for you? The student sitting in a lecture nodding and smiling at the lecturer, but really thinking 'What shall I wear to the club tonight'. The chattering child who receives a few 'mm' 'ahas' from her mum who is trying to read a magazine. The nervous interviewer who is trying to think of the next question, rather than listening to the answer to the last one. Have you had any similar experiences? On these sorts of occasions we are sometimes aware of what we are doing; at other times it is an unconscious action. It is only when we are caught out by someone asking us a question that we realise our lack of attention. Listening is a mental activity that requires effort and concentration.

Sometimes, although we think we have listened, our attitudes, preconceptions and prejudice distort the message. Here is an example of how assumptions about the client have prevented the doctor from 'hearing' the client's real concerns:

The doctor is treating the client for colitis (inflammation of the bowel). He is also aware that she is receiving treatment for another condition, endometriosis (this is sometimes, but not always discovered when a woman is being investigated for difficulty in conceiving). He has just informed her that she will have to continue to take her medication for colitis indefinitely.

CLIENT: I would like to try to come off the tablets and see what happens.

DOCTOR: It is important that you continue with the tablets. We know that any recurrence of the inflammation is usually worse.

CLIENT: I would still like to try.

DOCTOR: There is no need to worry if you are thinking about getting pregnant. We know that this type of drug has no effect.

CLIENT: I will stop the tablets for a few months and see what happens.

DOCTOR: That's up to you then.

The client's real concerns were not about getting pregnant, but the long term effects of taking the medication. The doctor had assumed from his knowledge of the client's medical history that she was anxious about having a baby. Look at the same situation with the doctor listening and responding to what the client is trying to say.

CLIENT: I would like to try to come off the tablets and see what happens.

DOCTOR: You would like to stop the medication. Are you having any problems with the tablets?

CLIENT: No. The tablets are okay. It's just that I don't like the idea of taking tablets for ever.

DOCTOR: You don't like the idea of staying on long term medication.

CLIENT: No. It can't do your body any good taking all this stuff all the time. And it's quite a drag carrying them round and making sure to take the dose.

DOCTOR: There are very few side effects with this drug. They usually show up fairly soon after people start taking them. You have no signs of any of these side effects, so you are unlikely to develop them in the future. However, we will be regularly monitoring you.

CLIENT: What happens if I stop taking them?

DOCTOR: We know that people usually have a flare up of the condition fairly quickly. Unfortunately the symptoms are usually worse. My advice is to continue with the medication.

CLIENT: I suppose I had better carry on taking them.

DOCTOR: We could try you on a reduced dose and see what happens.

CLIENT: Yes. I would like to try that.

He has followed the client's lead rather than imposing his own interpretation. By relating his verbal responses to the client he has shown that he has listened. This is another way of demonstrating to an interviewee that you are attending to what they are saying. Although the second exchange is longer, the client is far more likely to comply with the doctor's advice. The principle can be applied to any interview situation.

Here are some ideas of questions you can ask yourself to sharpen your listening skills:

- What is the person saying?
- Do you know why they are saying it?
- Are they consistent in what they are saying?
- How does what the person is saying compare with what you know already?
- What order do they say things? (This will give you some clues as to their priorities.)

○ Listen to how they say the message. Do they talk too quickly? Do they make themselves clear? Are they hesitant?

In observation, watching and listening are partners that complement each other. As you are listening, compare what you observe with what you are hearing. Is there any mismatch? For instance the client who says 'I'm fine' but looks in discomfort; or the appraisee who states 'I've got no worries about work', but looks concerned. These need to be noted and followed up.

Asking questions

Asking questions is one of the main ways by which we gather information. There are numerous types of questions that the interviewer can use. Some are distinguished by the type of response they elicit, and are categorised as closed or open.

The possible answers to a closed question are usually limited and require a short answer. The questioner sets the parameters for the answer, and therefore has more control over what the interviewee will say. 'Did you feel upset?' 'What was your previous salary?' 'How many children do you have?' are all examples of closed questions. These sorts of questions are often used on questionnaires.

In contrast, open questions allow the respondent to give a more elaborated response. Open questions usually start with 'Tell me about...' 'How did you...' 'Why did you...' These types of questions tend to be better at eliciting information about attitudes and opinions or encouraging the expression of feelings.

Another way of classifying questions is by function. The interviewer might use a number of different questions to make sure he understands the information the interviewee is giving. These are known as clarifying questions. So if the reply to a question is unclear, the interviewer might ask 'Do you mean that...' or 'Could you explain that again...' Asking for specific examples is another form of clarification.

There are some types of questions that interviewers need to avoid. They are:

Multiple questions (not to be confused with multiple-choice). This is when the interviewer asks several questions at once. An example is 'Where did you go to school? Was it near Exeter? You did go to school in this country didn't you?' These are difficult to answer and often confuse the interviewee. They must remember what you are asking and then formulate an answer for each one. Poor phrasing of a question the first time often leads to a multiple question as the interviewer tries to re-phrase his first attempt.

Leading questions. These are questions that 'lead' the person to the response that the interviewer would like to hear. So a question like 'You would agree that a driving licence is essential for this post' leaves the interviewee no choice but to agree.

The structure of your interview

There are various ways of structuring information gathering within the interview. These styles are linked to the type of questions used by the interviewer. The approach you choose will be determined partly by the purpose of the interview, and partly by your own personal approach to the situation. The main approaches to structuring information gathering are:

1. **The chronological approach.** Questions are asked in strict chronological order. In a selection interview the candidate would be asked questions on education, professional training and then subsequent employment until their current post. In a clinical interview a parent would be asked to relate details of the pregnancy, birth, early development and so on up to the current position. This approach provides the interviewer with a neat framework. However, it fails to address the individual, and therefore there is the possibility of omitting vital information or wasting time gathering unnecessary detail.

2. **Objective to subjective approach.** This approach organises information according to its emotional content. The interviewer starts with questions on topics that are not likely to produce anxiety or require much depth of thinking. Examples would be simple re-call questions like 'What is your date of birth?' 'When did you have your operation?' What passes did you obtain at 'A' levels?' As the interviewer establishes a rapport with the interviewee they progress to more subjective areas relating to feelings and attitudes. This type of approach is useful for situations where the interviewee is in a state of high emotional arousal. Examples would include disciplinary, grievance and some clinical interviews.

3. **Broad questions to specific questions.** In this approach the interviewer starts with open ended questions that are designed to encourage participation by the interviewee. For example, 'Tell me about your present post?' and 'How can I help you today?' These questions gradually become more specific or closed, like 'How

many people did you supervise?' and 'Does bending the knee hurt?' This style of interviewing places the focus on the interviewee. Questions are based on the information they provide, rather than the interviewer setting the agenda with their own questions. Some people are uncomfortable with this approach because control by the interviewer is reduced.

4. **Specific questions to broad questions.** This is the reverse of the above approach. The interviewer starts with a series of closed questions and graduates to more open ones. This is a useful if you want to relax the interviewer first with some simple questions. It also provides a way of establishing specific facts about the person.

Whatever the interview or the style of the interviewer, it is essential that the information gathering process has some sort of structure. This helps the interviewer who knows what he will ask and the way in which he will ask it. It also gives the interviewee a sense that the questioning has some purpose and direction. Any tendencies to jump from one topic to another and then back again are to be avoided. This sometimes happens with novice interviewers who are using a checklist approach. They may seek to go back over items they have missed. Or they are finding it difficult to make use of information provided by the interviewee because it does not match the order of their form.

Encouraging the interviewee

Good interviewing is an art. The successful interviewer is able to draw out information from the interviewee with the minimum of questions. This is achieved partly by the choice of question, and partly by encouraging contributions from the interviewee. We have already seen that open questions elicit longer replies. The way in which the interviewer responds to these replies will determine how much more the interviewee will say.

A simply pause after the interviewee has said something is often enough to elicit more information (Matarazzo *et al.* 1965). I once worked for a manager who used this technique with devastating effect. People divulged far more than they intended as they succumbed to the urge to fill the silences. These sorts of silences also signal to the interviewee that there is time and space for their views and opinions.

Other forms of encouragement are smiling, nodding and remarks like 'go on' and 'that's interesting'. The interviewee is more likely to respond at length if they receive these sorts of feedback. It shows that the interviewer is listening and interested in what they have to say.

There are other ways that the interviewer can demonstrate that he is listening. Asking questions related to what the interviewee has just said is a simple technique. Another more difficult method is repeating back the key points of the interviewee's response. This is discussed in more detail in the 'Clinical Interview' section.

Maintaining control over the interview

The opposite problem to the reticent interviewee is the overtalkative one. The discussion is taken over with the interviewer deluged by a verbal shower. The use of specific questions of the closed variety is one way of getting the interview back on track. The interviewer can also try reversing some of the non-verbal reinforcers used to encourage contributions. Talking about what you are doing also helps to slow down the pace. For example, 'I'm going to give you an example'. Some less sensitive individuals may need a direct statement telling them to keep their answers brief.

Clarification of information

Part of the process of gathering information is making sure you understand what you are being told. There are various ways of doing this. They include asking questions, requesting a repetition, asking for specific examples and summarising what you think has been said. It is important to check information as you go along. The interviewee is likely to become irritated if they find out you lost the thread of the discussion five minutes earlier.

Recording information

It is essential, and a legal requirement in the case of clinical notes, to make a written record of your discussions. Generally it is better to avoid writing whilst the interviewee is talking. You need to give them your full attention. In some interviews, notes can be made at the end.

The interviewee may need to see or have a copy of a summary of the interview. This is particular so in the case of appraisals, grievance and disciplinary.

Action Points

1. Practise this listening task with a friend. One person takes the role of the speaker, and the other is the listener. The speaker must talk for 2–3 minutes on a subject that interests them. The listener can ask questions, but must avoid giving any feedback like nodding or smiling. At the end the speaker should discuss how it felt.

   Repeat the activity, but this time the listener must provide lots of feedback. Compare the amount of talk between the two situations. Now swap roles so that you both have a turn at being the speaker.

2. Use this exercise to practice asking questions and to note the effects of different question forms. You will need an observer for this activity. Interview a friend about their hobby, favourite sport or a topic of their choice. Alternate between different question forms. The observer can use the checklist below to record the effects of your questioning. You may also like to see the effect of including a pause after the interviewee has responded.

Observation Sheet

	Responses			
	yes/no	few words	one sentence	several
Closed ?				
Open ?				
Multiple ?				
Leading ?				
pause				

3. Practise interviewing a friend using one of the methods for structuring information gathering discussed in the above section.

Summary Points

- Questionnaires, forms, historical information, specific recommendations and information from other agencies are all sources of information prior to the interview.

- Gathering information prior to the interview provides a focus for the discussion, and allows the interviewer to prepare more thoroughly. It also involves the interviewee in preparing and setting the agenda for the interview.

- Questionnaires and forms need to be available in a range of languages that reflect the cultural mix of the area.

- Interviewers need to be aware of any bias that might be created from information they receive about the interviewee, and that the actual information itself may be biased.

- The bulk of information gathering takes place during the interview.

- The interview situation provides the interviewer with the opportunity of observing the interviewee. Observation is about both watching and listening.

- It is important to create the right atmosphere for listening.

7

Involving the Interviewee

Involving the interviewee means increasing their control over the procedures and encouraging their participation. There are various ways of doing this throughout the interviewing process. They can be summarised as:

- Involving the interviewee in the arrangements for the interview
- Negotiating an agreed agenda
- Providing the opportunity for the interviewee to state their case
- Encouraging questions
- Providing information.

We have looked at most of these issues in *Setting the Scene* and *Gathering Information*. In this section I am going to concentrate on giving information. This is often a neglected area of the interview, but is a crucial aspect. For instance, Ley (1988) found that improving information giving to clients resulted in increased satisfaction with the interview.

What do we mean by information?

The type of information you will give is dependant on the context and the purpose of your interview. In a counselling interview the emphasis is likely to be about feelings and attitudes. An appraiser might want to discuss specific facts and figures.

The way that we give information will also vary. It might take the form of a report, an explanation or a set of instructions.

Barriers to effective information giving

Part of the skill in giving information is knowing what might interfere with the message. The first step is to identify the factors that affect communication.

Some of these can be eliminated. For example, noise makes it difficult to listen. The solution is to find a quiet interview room or take steps to get the noise stopped. Some factors need to be dealt with differently. The client who is distressed might find it very hard to assimilate what you are saying. It may be the message itself that is distressing the client, a poor prognosis or a diagnosis of disability. In this instance the message and the way the message is delivered will need to be altered. But the distress will still be there.

In any situation there are three main areas to consider:

○ The characteristics of the messenger
○ The characteristics of the receiver of that message
○ The context in which the message is sent.

The characteristics of the messenger

To give information in a coherent and comprehensive fashion, the messenger needs to have certain qualities. The principle qualification is an adequate knowledge. This is particularly pertinent to students or trainees who are in the process of acquiring knowledge. There is a difference between the level of understanding required to learn a subject, and the level required to explain the subject to someone else.

An effective communicator will also possess certain personal qualities. The ability to speak clearly is essential. Information needs to be presented at the right pace for the listener, and loud enough for him to hear. A fluent delivery is easier for the listener, than one full of hesitations and false starts. As well as having good oral skills, an effective communicator will be skilled in judging the needs of the listener – both in terms of the type and level of language required, but also in checking how much the listener is understanding and then modifying his message accordingly.

The effectiveness of our communication is also affected by how we are feeling. It is difficult to concentrate if we are tired, hungry or desperate for the loo. Changes in mood also alter our ability to interact with others.

The characteristics of the receiver

The intended message is not always the same as the one that is received. This is because of the individual characteristics of the receiver. Each of us varies in age, intelligence and personality. These characteristics affect our ability to receive and understand information. Because we all lead different lives we also have varied interests, experiences, expectations and attitudes to life.

People also vary on a day-to-day basis. They have mood changes. Their needs alter. Different stress points like admission to hospital or diagnostic tests will create anxiety (Corney 1991). All these factors affect the person's ability to listen to the message. For instance, they may only hear part of what you are saying because they have screened out the bad bits.

The context in which the message is sent

We all find it difficult to listen or converse if there are distractions. These can be extraneous noises, other people talking or the visual distraction of people walking pass the window.

Even the temperature of the room can affect how well we listen. A warm, stuffy room is likely to send us to sleep. We feel uncomfortable in a chilly room. The atmosphere and seating of a room all play a part in how well and for how long we can attend to a speaker. Think about the design of a fast food restaurant. Hard plastic seats and harsh lighting. The aim is to get a quick turn-over of customers. Compare this with the traditional country pub with log burning fire and cosy armchairs. The idea here is to keep the customers drinking for as long as possible.

Different types of information will alter the demands on our communication skills. Feelings and attitudes are harder to convey than facts and figures (Rees 1991). They may arouse strong emotions in both the interviewer and the interviewee. Emotionally loaded topics need careful wording.

Using appropriate language

Every time we speak we make a deliberate decision about what we are going to say, and a less conscious choice about how we are going to say it. When we speak to a child we use shorter sentences with simpler words – 'Did Daddy wave bye-bye?'. When we speak to an adult we generally use more complex utterances and a different vocabulary – 'Did your husband get the chance to say goodbye to you before he went?' In an interview we know that we have to adjust our language to the individual. We avoid jargon, slang or abbreviations, unless we know the person is familiar with them. The challenge is to select language that is appropriate to the individual. This is not always obvious. There is no simple equation.

Structuring your information

Before you can start to give any information you need to plan how you will present your material.

Select the key elements

One of the skills in giving information is knowing what you want to say and why you want to say it. This may seem an obvious point, but the rationale for giving information is sometimes overlooked. Inexperienced interviewers may choose information that demonstrates their knowledge or expertise. They are giving information for their own benefit, not the benefit of the interviewee.

The nature of your interview will dictate the type of information, but you will have to decide which are the key elements. Part of this decision will be based on how much and what type of information is required by the interviewee. This is a fine line. There is a danger of discriminating against individuals, because of your attitudes and beliefs about what they need to know. For example, if we omit to give older people information about safe sex. The ability to select appropriate material is an essential skill.

Avoid overloading

Individuals vary in the amount of information they can cope with at any one time. If you give too much information, the person will have difficulty in understanding and retaining the message.

Order your material

The order in which information is presented to the listener will affect their ability to understand and remember the message. When explaining it is important to start with the most important items and work your way through to the least important. We also know that it is difficult to understand the detail until we have the whole picture. So start with broad areas and gradually narrow these down to specific points (Shimoda 1994). For example, a therapist may advise a client with a voice problem that there are three things that she can do to improve her voice – relaxation, increasing fluid intake and avoiding shouting. These are the broad areas. The therapist may then go into specific details. So for increasing fluid intake she might describe why this is needed and how the client can achieve it. Some pieces of information have a natural sequence, such as procedures. Your description should follow this order.

Choose your words with care

The tone of your language will depend on the nature of your interview. Obviously a disciplinary hearing is very different from a selection interview. The words you use need to reflect the required tone. For instance, when your aim is to encourage the interviewee, you need to use positive words. King *et al.* (1983) suggest using 'when' instead of 'if' or 'try' (words that are associated with the possibility of failure).

Check your choice of words for ambiguity. The context will often make your message clear, even if your words are confusing. Look at these examples:

- Your mother is dying (*Doctor to the daughter*)
- Your mother is dyeing (*Art teacher to the daughter*)

- We need to examine your genes (*Doctor to his patient*)
- We need to examine your jeans (*Police officer to the suspect*)

Sometimes confusions arise in a completely unexpected fashion. The following conversation was overheard at a day hospital:

(The previous evening an unexploded bomb from the second world war had meant the local area had been evacuated. The doctor starts the interview with some friendly enquiries.)

DOCTOR: 'Were you evacuated yesterday?'

CLIENT: 'Yes, I open my bowels every day.'

The doctor had assumed the client would know about the bomb and the evacuation of the inhabitants. The client had expectations about what the doctor might ask. Bowel habits are always near the top of the list. A recipe for a comic mistake!

Whatever the interview, the participants need to make sure they share the same meanings for words. Otherwise the whole message becomes distorted.

Highlight Important Information

Help the listener to distinguish which parts of the message are important by emphasising key points. Use statements like 'This is a very important point...', to focus the attention of the listener. Reinforce the message non-verbally by slowing down and stressing key words.

Provide Explanations

Decide what type of explanation you need to give. (Brown 1978) identified three main types of explanation:

1. **Descriptive (how?)**

This type of explanation provides a straightforward description of structures, procedures and processes. For example, How is a smear test administered? How is a database set up?

2. **Interpretative (what?)**

   This type of explanation offers a definition of terms or seeks to clarify an issue. For example, What is oestrogen? What do the results of a blood test mean?

3. **Reason giving (why?)**

   This type of explanation attempts to give reasons. This often involves the discussion of principles, values and motives. For example, Why do I need a smear test? Why do women produce oestrogen?

Unless you are very experienced you will need to practise the skills of explaining. See the section on 'Lecturing' for more detailed information on planning an explanation.

Reinforce Your Message

Use as many channels as necessary to get your message across. Draw a diagram, use gestures or demonstrate with a model to help you convey exactly what you mean. Information is much more likely to be understood if the main points are repeated or summarised. This can be done intermittently during the interview, as well as at the end.

Checking the message has been understood

An essential component of giving information is checking how much has been understood. When we talk to our friends we are looking for signs and asking questions, to check that they understand what we are saying. If our friend looks confused or puzzled, we might ask 'I don't know if I am making myself clear, here?' In a similar way the interviewer uses non-verbal signals for feedback on how well her message is being understood, although care has to be exercised in interpreting some of these signals. A woman who had lost all ability to comprehend speech, convinced the doctor that she understood his questions by squeezing his hand at the appropriate moment. He had very obliging been holding her hand throughout the interview, and her reactions were purely emotional rather than a bona fide response.

Sometimes people consciously give out signals that they have understood, when in fact this is not the case. Have you ever been in a conversation where you were having difficulty understanding, but you nodded blankly at the speaker to save embarrassment? This is a common reaction from hearing people to the deaf. They encounter this so often that they have invented a sign to represent this phenomenon.

You can take steps to test how much the interviewee understands by asking them to repeat back what you have said. This has to be phrased appropriately, otherwise it may sound like 'repeat after me'. Phrases like, 'I am not sure I explained that very clearly, what points came across to you', will elicit a summary from the interviewee. The use of the word 'I' puts the onus on the interviewer, who then takes any responsibility for any misunderstandings (Hargie *et al.* 1994). In some interviews it may be more appropriate to make a straightforward request for a summary. For instance, in an appraisal the interviewer might ask the appraisee what he feels had been the most important points of the discussion.

Simple prompts like 'Is there anything else you would like to ask me?' or 'Do you have any questions?' encourage the interviewee to voice any unresolved queries. This is not a fail safe method. People are often inhibited about asking questions. This might be due to embarrassment, fear of appearing stupid or not wanting to waste your time.

Action Points

1. Think about instances in the past where you have been required to give information. How did you select the material? Which of the following reasons did it include?

   - to show off your superior knowledge
   - to validate your role as a professional
   - to increase somebody else's understanding
   - to offer support
   - to relieve anxiety
   - to make things clearer in your own mind.

2. Before your next interview prepare how you will give the interviewee information. Follow these steps:

   - Identify the key elements of your message
   - Decide on the most important pieces of information

- ○ Plan a structure for giving the information – most important first, broad areas then specific items
- ○ Think about how you will give the information (instruction, demonstration or explanation)
- ○ Check the words you intend to use for ambiguity or unnecessary jargon.

Practise giving the information to a friend. Ask them to repeat back the information. Have they understood the message? Were they able to identify the important parts of the message?

Summary Points

- ○ Involving the interviewee means increasing their control over the interview procedures and encouraging their participation.
- ○ Providing the interviewee with information helps to empower them.
- ○ There are different types of information including facts, figures, feelings, attitudes and opinions.
- ○ The way that we give information varies. It might take the form of a report, an explanation or a set of instructions.
- ○ The accuracy of the message is often affected by the characteristics of the sender, the receiver and the context in which the message is sent.
- ○ Adequate knowledge, clarity of expression and the ability to evaluate the listener's needs are essential skills in the effective communicator.
- ○ Each listener has individual characteristics that affect their ability to perceive the message. These include age, IQ, personality, expectations, attitudes and previous experiences.
- ○ Factors associated with the context, like distractions, atmosphere, seating and the subject matter also affect communication.

- Language and vocabulary need to be appropriate for the individual.
- Structure information by following these steps:
  - Identify key elements
  - Avoid overloading
  - Order material into a logical sequence
  - Avoid ambiguity
  - Set the tone by choosing appropriate words
  - Highlight important information
  - Structure explanations.
- Check the message has been understood. Use summaries, repetition, questions, or elicit a summary from the interviewee.
- Allow time for the interviewee to ask questions.

$\boxed{8}$

Completing the Interview

Bringing about the closure of an interview is a gradual process involving several stages. These include:

- Summarising
- Checking understanding
- Confirming decisions
- Planning future actions
- Acknowledging achievements
- Asking for questions
- Expressing appreciation
- Saying farewells.

As the interviewer you will initiate the completion of the topic under discussion, and follow some if not all the above stages. The nature and purpose of your interview will determine which ones are appropriate to your situation.

Time boundaries

The first step in planning the closure of your interview is setting your time boundaries to allow for a satisfactory closure. The time this will take will vary according to the purpose and nature of your interview. Obviously if a large amount of information has been exchanged, this stage of the interview will take longer. Alternatively you may want to spend some extra time on clarifying issues. Ideally you will have discussed with the interviewee the length of the meeting, but reminders about the time are still useful. For instance, 'In the last ten minutes I suggest...'

Summarising

A summary is a brief statement of the key points of the interview. These might be facts; figures; feelings; opinions; or problems that arose during the discussion. Summarising serves several functions:

- It consolidates the interviewee's understanding
- It aids retention of information
- It clarifies issues for the interviewee
- It makes the interviewer's expectations clear
- It helps establish a mutual understanding of what has been achieved.

Summarising is a skill that requires practice. It involves listening, understanding, memory, and expression. Although it is a competence usually associated with the completion of an interaction, it is part of a continual process that starts at the beginning of your interview. You need to listen and understand what the interviewee is saying. This information is stored, ready to be reproduced in your summary. However, before you can express the key points, you need to select relevant items of information. Once you have chosen the main points, you need to reproduce these in a succinct but coherent fashion.

Mini summaries can be provided during the main body of the interview. This will help to clarify issues for the interviewee before continuing with the discussion.

Checking understanding

Providing a summary is a useful technique. But there are some drawbacks. It gives you no feedback about how much the interviewee has understood, or how involved they are in what you are saying. If you combine a summary with asking questions, you make an active partner of the interviewee. The questions will require them to listen, as well as highlighting any misconceptions they might have. The interviewee also needs to have the opportunity to ask questions (Stewart and Cash 1988). Your aim is to establish a mutual understanding of what was discussed and what was achieved. You can then agree on the decisions.

Future plans

As part of the closure you need to give the interviewee information about what will happen in the future. In a selection interview this may be the date when a decision will be communicated to the candidate; for the client in a clinical interview it might be information about referral to other agencies. Sometimes a discussion or exchange is ongoing, and it would be inappropriate to terminate it at the end of the interview. Hargie *et al.* (1994) describe a type of closure they term 'motivational'; they suggest the use of statements designed to motivate the client in a particular course of action, or help them apply what has been discussed in the interview to a wider context. For example, a health visitor might suggest to a parent that the next time her child has a tantrum she try some of the behaviour techniques they have discussed. Sometimes these suggestions need to be more formalised. An example is the appraisal where individual objectives are set for the appraisee. It is important to keep a written record of any such commitments.

Goodbyes

The final part of your interview is the social ritual of 'saying your goodbyes'. This is the time to make some general remarks, which show your appreciation such as 'I've enjoyed meeting with you today', and social phrases like 'Have a good weekend.' It is important that what you say matches your non-verbal behaviour. If you look at your watch while saying 'I'm glad we had this talk', you are likely to offend or appear insincere. The way in which you end the meeting will affect how both participants will feel about meeting each other again. In a situation where there is an ongoing relationship, it is particularly important to maintain social niceties.

Action Points

1. One way of discovering how important closure is to our social relationships is to imagine a situation in which one of the stages is omitted. Think about an interview you have attended – it could be a selection interview, an appointment with your doctor, or your last appraisal. How would you have felt if one or more of these things happened:

   ○ The interviewer finished the discussion without any explanation.

   ○ The interviewer failed to summarise the main issues for you.

- ○ The interviewer failed to reiterate any commitments you had agreed to implement.

- ○ You were not asked if you had any questions.

- ○ You were not told what to expect next.

- ○ The interviewer failed to say goodbye.

2. Think about interviews where you have felt uncomfortable about how it ended. Can you identify what made you feel this way?

3. Practise summarising skills with a friend. Choose a television or radio programme that involves some sort of discussion. Both of you should listen, and then write down your own summaries of the main points. Compare your separate versions. Do they agree? Discuss how you selected points to include in your summary.

Summary Points

- ○ Closing an interview is a gradual process involving several different stages.

- ○ The nature and purpose of your interview will determine which stages are appropriate to your situation.

- ○ Plan your interviews to allow time for a satisfactory closure.

- ○ Providing a brief summary of the main points helps to consolidate and clarify information for the interviewee. It is an ongoing process throughout the interview, as it requires good listening and memory skills as well as the ability to recall relevant information.

- ○ Asking questions is a way of involving the interviewee in the summarising process, and helps to identify any misunderstandings.

- ○ Always allow some time for the interviewee to ask questions. This will help clear up any outstanding queries they might have about the discussion.

- ○ Future action needs to be discussed and agreed upon. A written record needs to be kept of these commitments.
- ○ The final part of the interview is the social rituals of saying goodbyes. This is the time for social remarks that help smooth the ending of the interview.

9

Dealing with Difficult Situations

Interviews give rise to difficult situations that present a challenge to our communication skills as both interviewer and interviewee. Our ability to cope with these specific situations stems from our knowledge, skills and previous experiences. Of these three, experience is the most valuable.

Consider the trepidation of the student when faced with a new set of circumstances, such as taking a case history for the first time. Often these are commonplace events to the clinician, who has had many opportunities to practise the relevant skills. Most important, the clinician has had the opportunity to discover how people react, and in turn develop a variety of responses. Dickson *et al.* (1989) describe these patterns of responses as schemas. They suggest that health professionals learn to develop a range of schemas that can be drawn upon in response to different contexts.

It is not only the student who is faced with difficult situations. A change in role, responsibilities or client group will bring new challenges for the clinician.

Developing coping mechanisms

Although there are many differences between situations, it is still possible to identify a common approach to developing coping mechanisms.

- The first step is to develop an awareness of the difficulties that might arise. This allows you the opportunity to prepare.

- Part of this preparation will involve trying to understand the motivations and needs of the other person. This will give you greater insight and tolerance.

- The core of your preparation will be the development of a set of responses or schemas to enable you to be flexible in your approach.

Each of these stages is looked at in detail below.

Difficulties for the interviewer

Here is a list of some of the difficult situations that may arise for the interviewer:

- Dealing with emotional states – anger, depression, distress, embarrassment
- Giving bad news – a poor prognosis, an unpleasant diagnosis, giving a reprimand
- Helping the interviewee cope with – bereavement, disability, poor work performance
- Coping with demanding communication situations – non-English speakers, clients with communication difficulties, the overtalkative or reticent client

Which of these situations have you experienced? Are there any other interviews you have found difficult that are not mentioned above? Think about what makes the situation difficult for you. Some common anxieties are:

> 'What do I do if I lose control of the interview?'

> 'I'm afraid of physical attack.'

> 'I know I'm suppose to be thinking about how the client feels, but how will I deal with my feelings?'

> 'It will be so embarrassing if I can't cope.'

> 'How can I tell someone, after twenty years of service, they have to go?'

> 'I hate having to deal with someone who is angry.'

> 'If I make a mistake will my supervisor think I'm stupid?'

Try to identify what your anxieties are in each of the situations.

Difficulties for the interviewee

It is useful to look at the same situations from the perspective of the interviewee. Imagine how you would feel in the following situations. If you have had similar experiences, try to think back to your emotions and reactions at the time.

- **Receiving bad news** – being disciplined, discovering you have a chronic illness, realising your child is disabled
- **Dealing with emotional states** – being afraid, suffering extreme anxiety, becoming irritated or angry
- **Coping with demanding communication situations** – not understanding, having difficulty in explaining, being embarrassed to ask questions

Understanding the motivation and needs of the other person helps increase our understanding, and therefore control over the situation. People are affected by:

- Previous experiences (mis-diagnosis, failed selection interviews)
- Previous relationships (particularly with authority figures)
- Physical state (pain, tiredness, hunger)
- Psychological state (depression, paranoia)
- Emotional state (distress, fear, anxiety)
- Situational factors (the amount of waiting time prior to the interview, opportunities for expressing their views)
- Personal circumstances (financial needs, aspirations, amount of support from friends and family)
- Personality (calm, out-going, reserved)

Look at these different scenarios. Which of the above factors are influencing the interviewee's reactions:

A young man has waited one and a half hours for his out-patient appointment. He was originally referred to the hospital eight months ago. He has recently started a new job, which requires heavy manual labour. Before this he was unemployed for eighteen months. His boss has allowed him time off for the appointment, but is docking his pay for the time he is not at work. When he finally sees the doctor he explodes in a rage when he is told that his back problem means he will have to spend six months in plaster and avoid any heavy lifting.

The mother of a seven-year-old child is insisting on a second opinion. She believes her child has a hearing loss. She has noticed that the child is a slow reader, and sometimes makes mistakes in her articulation. All tests so far have found the child's hearing to be normal. She has become increasingly depressed over the situation.

During a disciplinary interview, a manager becomes more and more irritated by the responses of the staff member. This person accompanies each statement with a laugh and a shrug of the shoulders. The manager finds it particularly difficult to understand their attitude, as they have known the individual for many years.

The district nurse is visiting a middle aged man who has just returned home from a hospital stay. He has had several months of intensive treatment for cancer. Unfortunately, this was unsuccessful. The implications of this were discussed with the man and his family before his discharge. He is discussing how well he feels with the nurse, and wondering why the hospital have arranged a Macmillan nurse. He then goes on to describe his holiday plans for next year.

Developing schemas

The development of schemas is a learning process, and can be approached in the same way as any other learning situation.

Read around on the appropriate subject matter. For instance, in the case of bereavement it is useful to find out about the stages of grief through which people pass. Without this sort of information you may find the person's behaviour odd or unexpected.

If possible observe other people in similar situations. Note both what they are saying and how they are saying it. Check the reactions of the other person. Is what the person saying effective? Remember to look at non-verbal communication and paralinguistic features, such as posture and tone of voice. How are silences used?

Think about previous experiences. What did you learn that could help you in the present situation? Use the action points to help you draw upon previous experiences. More information is provided on dealing with specific situations in the *interviews in context* section.

Action Points

Try these activities with a friend or colleague. The imaginary situations do not necessarily have to be a formal interview, as these activities focus on feelings, reactions and coping mechanisms in general.

1. Describe a difficult situation that you have dealt with successfully to your partner. Discuss how you coped with it. Now listen to your partner as they describe a situation.

2. Think of situations you found difficult as a student. How did you cope? What are your reactions to similar situations now? (If you are presently a student, think back to your early experiences on practical placement or to situations you have dealt with in the past.)

3. Identify a new challenging situation that occurred recently. This might be at work, home or in a social situation. Choose one you felt you dealt with successfully. What was new about the situation for you? *A different role? A new experience? A change in circumstances?* What experiences did you draw upon to deal with it? Would you deal with it differently now?

   Try the following exercise with a group of people. (The above exercises can also be used by a group. People can pair off and then return to the larger group to discuss their ideas.)

4. A common situation is chosen by the group. Each person describes one strategy they have used to cope with a similar situation. They should try to link this with a personal quality they possess such as 'good listener' or 'knowledge of a certain subject'.

Summary Points

- Our knowledge, skills and previous experiences help us to cope with difficult situations.

- Experience is the most valuable asset.

- Health professionals learn to develop a set of responses or schemas that enable them to take a flexible approach.

- Increasing our awareness of the difficulties we might face allows us the opportunity to prepare.

- By understanding the motivations and needs of the other person, we well have greater insight and tolerance.

- The development of schemas is a learning process.

- Read around the appropriate subject area.

- If possible observe other people in similar situations.

10

Working with Interpreters

This section provides information and guidelines about working with interpreters during a clinical interview.

Why do you need interpreters?

Interpretation ensures equal access to health care and health information for persons whose first language is not English. It enables these clients to discuss their health needs in depth, and to make informed choices about their treatment and care. They can also express anxieties or concerns regarding test procedures and treatment. For the health professional improved communication with the client will assist in diagnosis and treatment, and be beneficial to the relationship with the client in general.

When do you need interpreters?

It is difficult to give precise criteria for identifying clients who require the services of an interpreter. You will have to make a judgement about this based on how well you think the client understands English, and whether they are able to express their needs adequately. Remember some people may be reluctant to reveal a language difficulty.

It is impossible to have an interpreter available for every conversation between the client and a health worker, for instance, on a daily basis on the ward. However, there are situations where interpretation is essential. These include:

- taking a case history from the client
- obtaining information for assessment purposes
- explaining the purpose of test procedures
- describing test procedures
- giving instructions during test procedures

- giving the client information on diagnosis and prognosis
- giving the results of test procedures
- prescribing treatment.

Who are 'interpreters'?

An interpreter is a person who is fluent in at least two languages. However, interpreting is not just about being multilingual. An interpreter will have undergone a specific training in the strategies and processes of interpreting. They will be a professional, and adhere to a code of practice. The work of an interpreter is not voluntary, although payment for interpreting services may be made by a voluntary organisation.

What does an interpreter do?

The interpreter's role is to interpret messages between yourself and the client by translating one language into a second language. The Council for the Advancement of Communication with Deaf People (CACDP) provide a succinct description for sign interpretation – 'the interpretation process involves expressing the same meaning and intent in a different vocabulary and grammatical structure'. This definition applies just as aptly to oral language interpretation.

The role of the interpreter does not go beyond the translation aspect. They are unlikely to know your client personally or know anything about their background or circumstances. They are not an expert on the culture of the client.

Why do I need a professional interpreter?

It is commonplace to find family members, often children, being used to interpret in a health setting. There are a number of difficulties with this situation, not least the lack of privacy and confidentiality for the client. One major issue is that you have no way of knowing the fluency of this 'interpreter', and therefore the accuracy of the information that is elicited or conveyed.

There is also the added dimension that the participants have a personal relationship. The family dynamics may interfere with the interviewing process considerably. There may be a reluctance to discuss certain issues or convey bad news. Personal questions may cause embarrassment among family members.

Acceptance or attitudes to different medical conditions may vary or influence what and how the message is translated. Issues of birth control, sexually transmitted diseases, disability and other less predictable subjects are areas that arouse strong feelings. The family member may give their own views, which could be confused as medical advice by the client.

Bilingual health professionals are often encouraged to volunteer their services as interpreters. There are problems with this approach, some of them similar to those found when using family members.

Health workers may also create confusion for the client by adopting two roles. This is particularly pertinent to those health workers who are already involved with the client's care. Is the worker addressing them as the health professional or an interpreter?

The family member or volunteer health professional will have no training in the strategies and processes of interpreting. Information relevant to a diagnosis may be omitted or altered by the failure to interpret the message literally. For example, failing to translate the confused nature of speech in the client with dementia, or using general terms rather than specific ones, such as 'pain' when the response was 'cramp'.

What are the responsibilities of the health professional?

The ultimate responsibility for the interview lies with the health professional. This includes:

○ providing the interpreter with all the information necessary to carry out the assignment

○ explaining terminology to the client

○ answering questions from the client

○ providing the client with explanations

○ making sure the client has understood

○ giving instructions to the client.

What are the responsibilities of the interpreter?

The interpreter is a professional who will adhere to a code of practice. You can expect the interpreter to:

○ be competent

○ be fluent in receiving and expressing messages in both the language of the interviewer and the language of the client

○ refuse work that is beyond their capabilities

- ○ maintain client confidentiality
- ○ follow a code of ethics
- ○ be professional in their approach to the situation and the client
- ○ respect the boundaries of their role. An interpreter will not offer the client advice or proffer their opinions on either the subject under discussion or on the health professional.
- ○ remain impartial
- ○ not use information for their own personal use or gain.

How does the communication context change?

The interaction in an interpreted interview differs significantly from the normal situation in a number of ways. Questions and responses are repeated as they are interpreted from one language to another. Occasionally the interpreter will ask you or the client to repeat a question or they may be unsure of the exact meaning of a statement. This results in a longer time between turns at speaking, and a slower pace. This means that the interview will usually take longer than normal.

Turn-taking needs to be established from the beginning of the interview. This means one person speaking at a time. The interpreter can only concentrate on one message.

In a clinical interview important information for the health professional is often obtained through observing the client. Attitudes might be revealed by the way a client phrases a statement, or anxiety signalled by the client hesitating before asking a question. A professional interpreter will interpret everything and try to express any nuances in the communication. However, it is important still to watch out for these non-verbal clues, even when it is the interpreter talking to the client.

Despite these differences your communication style will not differ from that of any other interview. It is your responsibility to make sure that the client has understood and to offer explanations as appropriate. The client must also have the opportunity to ask questions and query treatment options.

How does it affect the client?

The personal nature of interviews in the health context require that the situation is handled carefully and with sensitivity. The client may feel embarrassed about their health problems or the intimate nature of examinations and test procedures. They may be reluctant to discuss certain symptoms and illnesses, particular those that are seen as less socially acceptable. The addition of a third person into this setting can increase the stress for the client.

The relationship between the client and the interpreter will affect the amount and quality of the information you obtain. It is important to be aware of any potential barriers to the formation of an effective relationship. Two obvious factors are the gender and age of the interpreter. Generally a same sex interpreter is the ideal choice. Age may also be an issue. Some clients may prefer someone of around the same age, whilst others may feel more comfortable with someone older or younger than themselves. Attitudes to certain issues differ between generations, for example sex before marriage. A professional interpreter would not allow personal opinion to affect their work, but a client may feel the interpreter is making a judgement or has a particular view.

Cultural and social background is another area that may create difficulties; for example, the difference between an Asian person born in England and one from the subcontinent. Ask for an interpreter with the same culture and background as your client.

Interpreters familiar with working in the health care context will be aware of the special demands of this situation. They will assist the interviewer by responding professionally. If necessary, the interpreter can stand behind a screen or leave the room to allow the client some privacy. In these circumstances all instructions need to be given prior to the interpreter leaving the room, and no new information can be given until they return. In all cases, except in certain mental health cases, the clients have the right to refuse an interpreter.

Guidelines for working with an interpreter

- Book the interpreter well ahead of the interview. Use the checklist at the end of this section to make sure you have given all the relevant details.
- Check that the interpreter is able to speak the dialect your client is using, and whether the gender, age or background of the interpreter might cause discomfort to the client.
- Give the interpreter complicated information, including technical terms, in advance so they can prepare themselves.
- Alert the interpreter to any special procedures you might be using.

- ○ Allow time before the interview to discuss the purpose and nature of the interview. Check that the interpreter is clear about their role and the extent of their involvement in the interview.
- ○ Give the interpreter an opportunity to establish a rapport with the client before the interview.
- ○ During the interview look at the client and not the interpreter. Refer to the client directly, not through the interpreter. For example, 'Do you get indigestion?' is preferable to 'Ask him if gets indigestion?' or 'Does he get indigestion?'.
- ○ Remember the interpreter has to mentally process information. Break your communication down into manageable chunks. Ask one question at a time and when giving information restrict it to two or three sentences at a time.
- ○ The interpreter can only attend to one message at a time. Avoid making conversational asides to colleagues. When there are several family members attending the interview it will be necessary to establish some ground rules about turn-taking.
- ○ Do not expect too much of the interpreter. Interpreting is a demanding task. There is no rest between questions and answers as with normal conversations. Therefore you need to be aware of how much you are asking the interpreter to do and for how long. The optimum time is twenty minutes with occasional breaks. Anything longer than two hours needs more than one interpreter.

Interpreters for the sensory impaired

Sensory impairment refers to individuals who have impairment of either their vision or their hearing, or both. Interpretation is usually required by individuals who are deaf or deaf–blind. The type of interpretation required by these two groups varies both between and within the two groups. An understanding of the different modes of communication will help you in working effectively with interpreters and the sensory impaired.

Deaf people

Deaf people born with, or acquiring a profound hearing loss within the first few years of life are likely to communicate through British Sign Language or Sign Supporting English.

British Sign Language (BSL) British Sign Language can be defined as 'a visual-gestural language' (Deuchar 1984), and is the natural language of many deaf people in Britain. Meaning is expressed through the use of signs produced by movement of the hands and arms; facial expression including lip patterns; and movements of the head and body. Unlike oral languages, which rely on the auditory channel, BSL uses vision. Some lip patterns are used, but words are never spoken. Although it appears to be mime or elaborate gesture, it is in fact a language with its own distinct grammar. Sign languages are not universal, so American Sign Language is different from British Sign Language.

Signs Supporting English (SSE) Spoken English is accompanied by the use of signs, usually supporting key words in the sentence. The structure of sentences will follow English word order and grammatical rules. Speech is usually used with the signs. Many deaf BSL users will convert to a form of SSE when communicating with hearing people who have limited sign abilities.

Finger Spelling Finger shapes and patterns of hand movements are used to represent the 26 letters of the English alphabet. Words can be spelt out using the alphabet. Some signs consist of a fingerspelling pattern where a few letters represent a word, for example 'father' is signed by fingerspelling 'f' twice. Fingerspelling is used by both BSL and SSE signers. Unusual medical terms are more likely to be expressed by finger spelling than through signs.

Partially hearing and hard-of-hearing people
Partially hearing or hard-of-hearing people born with or acquiring a hearing loss later in life may not be signers, but may still require some assistance from lipspeakers or note takers.

Lipspeakers A lipspeaker repeats what the interviewer is saying to the deaf person, but mouths the words without using their voice. Lipspeakers are specially trained in communication skills, and are easier for the deaf person to lip-read. The information is conveyed as accurately as possible, but occasionally the lipspeaker may need to paraphrase a message that is too fast to lip-read. A lipspeaker is often required when the lipreader is meeting with more than one person.

Note takers This is a person who records the message verbatim in written form. There are a number of technical devices designed specifically for this purpose. The note taker types in the message, which appears on a screen for the deaf person to read.

Deaf–blind

The deaf–blind person may be unable to use the auditory or visual channels for communication. The deaf–blind manual alphabet is one method of communication that relies on the sense of touch. This is the method most likely to be used by the interpreter.

Deaf–Blind Manual Alphabet This is similar to the fingerspelling alphabet of the deaf, except that the shapes and patterns of the hand movements have been adapted to be tactile rather than visual. The interpreter spells out letters on the hand of the receiver using different parts of the hand and different strokes to represent the letters. For example the index finger laid across the palm of the receiver indicates an 'I'.

Working with interpreters for the sensory impaired

When obtaining an interpreter for a deaf person it is essential to establish what type of interpretation they require. Signers need to state their preference for British Sign Language, Sign Supporting English, lipspeakers and so on. An appropriate interpreter can then be allocated. Remember that not all deaf people are signers or need interpretation. Ask first, before you make any arrangements.

Visual materials, models and drawings can be used to help when explaining to a deaf person. Remember to let the deaf person look at the visual information before you discuss it. It is not possible to follow signing or lip-read if you are looking at something else, like a picture or a drawing.

Sign interpreters

Sign language interpreters communicate using a visual system, and therefore positioning is crucial. They need to see, and be seen by the deaf client. Ask the interpreter where they would prefer to sit before you start your interview. Below are some guidelines on positioning which will help you to anticipate some of their needs.

Aim to seat the interpreter:

- so light falls on their face
- facing the deaf person, preferably to one side of the interviewer so they are both in the client's sightline
- two or three metres away from the deaf person

- against an uncluttered background

Avoid seating the interpreter:

- in front of a window so that the light source is behind them and their face is in shadow
- in front of a cluttered notice board
- a busy background with people passing to and fro.

Manual language interpreter

The interpreter needs to be seated in a position where they can comfortably reach the client's hand. This is usually alongside the client.

Summary Points

- Interpretation helps all clients to have equal access to health care.
- Interpreters:
    - have undergone a specific training
    - are a member of a professional body
    - adhere to a code of practice
    - adhere to a code of ethics
    - are fluent in at least two languages.
- Avoid using non-professional interpreters. They may lack the high level of language skills required and omit or alter important information. They will have no training in professional ethics.
- Interpretation is needed when obtaining information for case history and assessment, explaining procedures, giving information about test results and prescribing treatment.
- The ultimate responsibility for the interview lies with the health professional. This includes providing the interpreter with the necessary information; and explaining and answering questions from the client.

- The interpreter will execute his or her responsibilities according to their code of practice, which includes ethical behaviour and maintaining client confidentiality.

- Interpreted interviews have a slower pace and participants need to agree on a routine for turn-taking.

- It is important that the interpreter and client are able to develop a comfortable relationship. Any potential difficulties such as gender or cultural differences need to be identified before the interview.

- Individuals who have a sensory impairment may need interpreting services. Ask the client if they require interpreting services. Check which type of interpretation they require.

- Book interpreters well in advance and provide them with as much information as possible.

Checklist for Booking an Interpreter

Book interpreters several weeks in advance, and confirm the details in writing. Give the interpreter as much information as possible. If you are flexible about times and dates you are more likely to find one available.

Check you have provided these basic details:

Interview Details

☐ Have you stated where the interview will take place?

☐ Does the interpreter know the date and time?

☐ Have you stated an estimate of the length of the interview?

☐ Have you given details of the nature and subject matter of interview?

☐ Is the interpreter clear about their role and the extent of their involvement in the interview?

☐ Have you given the name(s) of the interviewer(s)?

Client Details

☐ Have you given the interpreter the name, age and gender of the client or clients?

☐ Have you provided information about the client's ethnic background?

☐ Does the interpreter know the language of the client?

☐ Have you stated the dialect of the client?

Is there any other relevant information the interpreter needs to know?

- -

Name of interpreter:_____

Telephone Number:_____

Contact address:

_____

_____

_____

☐ Does the interpreter know how to contact the interviewer?

Date information sent:_____

Interviewing Skills in Context
Clinical Interviews

The clinical interview is the main point of contact with the client. It might take place in the clinic, on the ward or in the client's home. The purpose of the interview will depend on the needs of the client, and the action that has taken place to date.

An initial interview will focus on gathering information about the nature and development of the client's problem. This will help in forming a diagnosis and if possible identifying causative factors. This information forms the client's case history, which is recorded in their notes.

Some of the information contained within this case history will assist the clinician in formulating a therapeutic plan. For instance, factors that are contributing to the maintenance of a problem will need to be tackled. Treatment will also be affected by the amount of support available to the client.

The clinical interview is itself a therapeutic medium. The client is able to discuss his anxieties and concerns. In response the clinician can offer emotional support and care. It is the interview that helps to establish and maintain this relationship.

This section looks at strategies and techniques that can be used to increase the effectiveness of the clinical interview. Like any other interview, the first step is preparation.

Preparation

Gather any relevant material. This will include referral letters, reports from other agencies, previous records and the results of any investigations. Read these as thoroughly as time allows, asking yourself the following questions. What has happened to the client in the past? What is happening to the client now? Why were they referred to you?

This will help you to determine what you want to achieve from the interview. Is it assessment? Do you want to discuss the results of recent investigations? Make a plan for the interview, but be ready to modify this according to needs of the client (Clare 1991).

Setting the scene

Waiting room

It is not always possible to plan waiting areas in the way that you desire, because of cost restrictions and limitations due to shared accommodation. This is unfortunate as they set an important first impression.

One simple adaptation is to change the arrangement of the chairs. These are often placed in formal rows that face in one direction, or are positioned around the walls of the room. A friendly atmosphere is created by grouping some of the chairs in small circles, so that people have the opportunity to talk to each other.

The waiting room is the obvious place for posters and leaflets that promote health awareness in the client. Do you make the most of this opportunity?

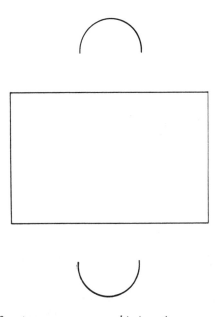

Figure 2.1a Types of seating arrangements used in interviews

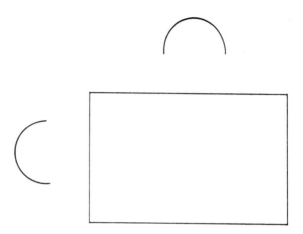

Figure 2.1b Types of seating arrangements used in interviews

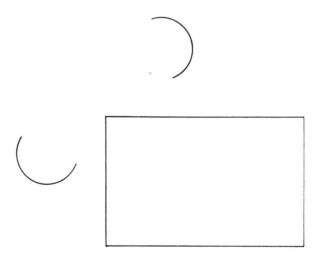

Figure 2.1c Types of seating arrangements used in interviews

Clinic room

The arrangement of chairs is just as important in the clinic room. Cook (1970) found that people preferred to sit at right angles to each other for conversation, as opposed to directly opposite. This set up can be replicated in the clinic. Make sure that you are facing towards the client. Figure 2.1 compares different arrangements.

- ○ Position (a) is confrontational and has an air of formality.

- Position (b) is better, but the clinician is still facing away from the client.
- Position (c) is a much more relaxed arrangement. The clinician and the client are facing each other.

Remember to re-arrange chairs after any interviews that involve several people. Otherwise the next client will be faced with an array of empty chairs left by the previous occupants. This avoids any confusion for the client about where they should sit.

The other main consideration about the clinic room is privacy. The client will be inhibited from discussing personal issues if they think they can be overheard. Unfortunately many rooms seem to lack any basic soundproofing. Soft furnishings such as carpets and curtains help, but are not appropriate in many clinical situations. Increasing the noise level in the waiting room is one way of masking out any sounds that come from the clinic room. Piped background music is an option, or installing a video playback facility. The latter could be used to show health promotion videos, cost and security allowing.

You can help by being aware of the problem, and being careful to restrict personal discussions wherever possible to private areas. In some situations, such as on a hospital ward, it is very difficult to achieve privacy. In these circumstances you will have to use side rooms or at the very minimum pull the curtains around the bed.

Establishing a rapport with the client

Your relationship with the client is an essential element of the interview (Clare 1991). You need to establish a rapport with the client as soon as possible. This will encourage him to be co-operative and develop his confidence and trust in you as a professional. There are a number of ways of achieving rapport.

Greetings

It is important to get the interview off to a good start, as clients form an impression within the first few minutes (Thompson 1984). At first greet the client by their full name until you have established their preferred form of address. Some clients like to be called by their first names. Other people find the use of their full name and title more acceptable.

Introductions

The focus of the clinical interview is the client, so it is easy to forget to tell him something about yourself. At the beginning of the interview introduce yourself to the client using your name and job title. Give a brief description of your role in non-professional terms that the client will understand.

A reference needs to be made to the referring agent in your introduction. For example, 'Dr Yu has asked me to see your child about his movement and balance'. This helps to set the interview in context, and demonstrates that you have read the referral information (Newell 1994).

Setting an agenda

You need to explain the purpose of the interview to the client. What are your intentions regarding the interview? Is it diagnostic? To provide treatment? Find out the intentions of the client. What do they want from the interview? A sick certificate? Information? The cause of their illness? Any mismatch is likely to cause misunderstandings and annoyance. Make it clear to the client if you are unable to fulfil any of their expectations. For instance, if you need to refer the client to other agencies.

Non-verbal communication

Body posture and gaze have been found to be significant in expressing rapport. A study by Harrigan *et al.* (1985) found that doctors who faced their clients, leaned forwards, sat closer and kept their arms and legs in an open position were perceived as having a high rapport. Those who sat farther away in an erect position or leaning back with asymmetrical arm and leg positions were perceived as having less rapport.

Empathy

An essential personal quality required by the health professional is the ability to have empathy for the client. This is about being able to take the client's perspective and understand how they might be feeling (Porritt 1984). It is distinct from feelings of sympathy. This is when you experience the feelings you yourself would have felt in a similar situation to the client (Gask 1991).

If you can convey empathy to the client, he is more likely to feel reassured and understood. One way of doing this is by showing the client you are attending to them. Use eye-contact, facial expression and head nods to show you are interested in the client and the client's problem. These non-verbal signals coupled with a warm, friendly tone will encourage the client to make contributions to the discussion (Huntington 1987).

Reflecting is another way of showing you have listened and understood. This is a technique borrowed from counselling, which can also be of use in the general interview situation. Look at these two examples of reflection:

The clinician is talking to a young adult stammerer.

(1) CLIENT: 'I've had two or three jobs in catering. I worked at the biscuit factory for a while. After that I did some sewing work at home. I'm not working at the moment though.'

CLINICIAN: 'You've had a wide variety of work experience.'

(2) CLIENT: 'Oh, I don't go out much. I'd like to go out and meet people some more. Sometimes I stay in every evening and all weekend. At times I feel quite desperate.'

CLINICIAN: 'It sounds as if you feel very lonely.'

The responses of the clinician reflect the essence of the client's message. However, they are not a simple repetition. The clinician uses her own words to express her understanding of what the client has said. In the first example the clinician deals with facts as they are presented by the client. In the second example the clinician is concentrating on the client's feelings.

Reflecting needs to be used with care, particularly when dealing with feelings. It is very easy to transpose your own feelings and reactions to the client. This comes back to the idea of sympathy as opposed to empathy. Interpretation of feelings must be approached with caution. Despite this it is a very effective interviewing technique.

Eliciting information from the client

One of the main aims of the clinical interview is to gather information. This information has to be relevant, accurate and as complete as possible. Before the clinician starts asking questions she needs to listen.

Listening

Burnard (1992) makes the point that we need to be attending to the client before we can truly listen to them. He describes three domains of attention. These are attending out, attending in and attending to fantasy. The first is when we focus our attention on external events and people. In the clinical interview this would be the client. The second refers to the attention we pay to our own thoughts and feelings. We are looking in on ourselves. The third refers to the internal dialogue that we sometimes have with ourselves. Pondering over possible interpretations of the client's words is one example of this type of attention. Using this model it is easy to see how difficulties can arise with listening.

Effective listening involves focusing on the client, or attending out, as Burnard describes it. This means concentrating on the information presented by the client and not on the process of data collection. Avoid using a set list of questions; instead let the client lead the discussion.

The structure of the interview

The first point to establish in the interview is why the client is attending (Pendleton *et al.* 1984). Use open ended questions (Cohen-Cole and Bird 1991) to encourage the client to tell you about the problem. Listen to what is of importance for the client. How does he describe the problem? What does he think caused the problem? Note the associations the client makes between ideas, and how he prioritises the information he gives.

By allowing the client to present his story of events you immediately involve him in the assessment. This will clearly indicate to him that his views are valued. It also gives him the chance to express any fears and concerns. Some clients will need to talk through their feelings early on in the interview. Others may feel uncomfortable with this approach, preferring to follow the lead of the clinician.

Once the client has given you some information, you can follow this up with more specific questions. Prepare the client by describing the type of information you need to know, and providing a brief explanation of the purpose of your questions.

Questions

Students often equate the case history with a checklist of questions. In fact questions are just one of the tools used by the clinician to gather relevant information. Questions should be prompted by what the client is saying, rather than being pre set.

You can check the appropriateness of your questions by asking yourself the following: Why are you asking this question? How do your questions relate to each other? How do your questions relate to the problem? It is best to avoid:

(1) Eliciting yes/no responses

Unless you are clarifying information, these should normally be avoided. They give you very little information. Compare the responses you would receive from these two questions:

'Has Viet been immunised?'

'What vaccinations has Viet had?'

(2) Appearing judgmental

The way that you phrase a question may indicate a certain opinion or bias. A parent who is asked: 'You didn't smack him did you when he wet the bed' is unlikely to feel confidant about revealing any other methods of disciplining the child. A question like 'What do you do when he wets the bed' is better.

(3) Asking leading questions

Avoid leading the client to what you think will be the likely answer. For example, 'You must be worried about the treatment?' Let the client express how they are feeling.

Keeping control of the interview

The novice interviewer probably worries most about maintaining control over the interview. Sometimes the client may wander off the topic. You need to bring them gently back to the point. Always make sure you acknowledge what they are saying first. 'Yes, that's interesting' or 'I see what you mean'. Then draw them back to the original topic. Phrases like 'You were saying before that...' and 'I would like to find out more about what you said earlier' will reinstate the original subject matter. Remember that using closed questions is one way of focusing the interviewee.

Checking on accuracy

Research has found that the diagnosis could have been made from the case history alone in many cases seen by doctors (Hampton *et al.* 1975; Myerscough 1989). There is no doubt that the case history is a useful evaluative tool for all health professionals. However, the value of this material is directly related to its accuracy.

Because of the historical or reported information contained in case histories, it has a natural tendency towards inaccuracy. The main difficulty is related to memory. The client may be willing to provide the information, but is unable to remember the details. Another common problem is that the client or family have developed a 'story' to account for the problem. For example, a swarm of gnats causing ulceration of the legs, even though the two events were quite separate. The facts become distorted to fit in with the family's theory. The skilled clinician is able to help the client remember and improve the accuracy of their responses by using a variety of strategies. The most common are:

(1) Asking for examples

This is useful to check the client's understanding of a particular term, or to encourage them to be more specific. For example 'What do you do when you feel anxious?' or 'Can you give me an example of the types of instructions Jay can now understand?'

(2) Asking for reasons

This will help establish why the person has come to a particular conclusion. For example, 'What makes you think he has a hearing loss'.

(3) Using clarification questions

These questions ask the client to explain a statement. For example, 'What do you mean when you say...?' or 'Are you saying...?'

(4) Using suggestions

Sometimes a client may find it difficult to put the answer into words. The clinician can suggest some possible responses. For example, 'What colour was the blood in your stools? – bright red, dark red...'. This method has to be used with care as it is easy to put words into the client's mouth.

(5) Establishing exact dates

Clients often group events together in their memory. Ask for specific dates to determine the exact sequence of events.

(6) Using memory joggers

The client may be able to remember when one event occurred by relating it to another. This often triggers off a whole series of memories. You can try this yourself by thinking of an important event like leaving school or a special birthday. What other things have you remembered?

(7) Using mini summaries

The clinician summarises what the client has said, who then has the opportunity to correct any misunderstandings.

The case history

A case history documents the discussions between the client and the health professional. It serves a number of purposes that include the following:

- ○ To act as documentary evidence of contact with a specific client
- ○ To record information relevant to the health care of the client
- ○ To focus subsequent clinical examinations and investigations
- ○ To provide a systematic way of organising information
- ○ To facilitate continuity of care.

The information contained within a case history helps the clinician in making a diagnosis and establishing the needs of the client in terms of therapy or treatment. For children, it also provides a description of developmental and behavioural patterns over time (Cohen 1983).

Below are examples of adult and paediatric case histories. These are in the form of guides that suggest areas where the clinician needs to direct their information gathering.

These are general guidelines only, as each discipline will vary in the amount and type of information required. For example, a full account of employment may be required from a client with a respiratory problem; whereas a full social history might have greater significance for a client presenting with mental health problems.

Examples of specific questions have been avoided, as the type and style of question will vary according to the needs and responses of the client.

Adult case history

Identification details

- ○ Name
- ○ Address
- ○ Telephone number
- ○ Date of birth and age
- ○ Client's identification number
- ○ Form of address preferred by the client (first name; title – Mr. Misses, etc.)
- ○ Name and address of next of kin.

Administrative details

- ○ Date of the interview
- ○ Place of the interview
- ○ Name and designation of the interviewer.

Referral information
- ○ Name and designation of the referring agent.
- ○ Reason for the referral/admission.
- ○ Date of the referral.

Nature of the problem
- ○ A description of the symptoms
- ○ Date when the problem first started
- ○ The way in which it first became apparent to the client.

Record a description of the problem using the client's words.

History of the problem
- ○ Development of the problem

    Establish whether the problem has changed in character or severity. Note any circumstances that are associated with these changes.

- ○ Consistency of the problem

    Note any times when the problem is better or worse; and any conditions associated with these periods.

Write a clear record of the development of the problem in chronological order. The onset and sequence of symptoms need to be dated as accurately as possible.

Effect on client

Note how the problem is affecting the client and the family. (Relationships; financially; socially; as well as physical effects such as fatigue, etc.)

Client's attitude to the problem

This section deals with information on the feelings and attitude of the client and family towards the problem, and about the referral itself.

Previous history of assessment

This section refers to previous investigations of the current problem. Find out where the client was seen before, and the name of the professional who dealt with the case. The results of these investigations need to be obtained.

Previous history of treatment

This section refers to the details of previous treatment relevant to the current problem. Find out the place of treatment and the name of the clinician.

- Note information about the type, length and purpose of the previous treatment
- Establish whether the client is currently receiving treatment elsewhere
- Reasons for a second referral need to be investigated and recorded.

Social history

FAMILY HISTORY

- *Parents* – Note information about age, occupation and general health. If deceased, note the age at time of death, and the cause of death.
- *Siblings* – Note their names, ages and position in the family. Details on marital status and occupation may also be required in some circumstances.

Enquire about any family history of illness or disability.

PERSONAL HISTORY

- Find out who lives with the client, and their relationship to the client
- Note the name, age and occupation of the client's partner or spouse
- Note the names, ages and occupation of any children
- Educational history may be appropriate in some circumstances.

Employment history

- Client's present or previous occupation. (A full record of employment history may be required in some cases.)
- Client's views regarding the effect of the problem on their occupation or employment prospects.

Habits

- ○ Quantity and frequency of smoking or drinking.
- ○ Eating habits including diet and appetite.
- ○ Sleeping habits including any recent disturbances to the client's usual routine.

Medical history

- ○ Periods of hospitalisation with the place, dates and reason for admission
- ○ Details of surgical procedures. (The place where they were performed and the outcome.)
- ○ Major illness or accidents
- ○ Results of relevant tests.

Record major events in chronological order with the details of the date, circumstances and outcome of each episode.

Current health status

- ○ Current health status of the client. Note details of menstruation and contraception in women.
- ○ *Medication* – Record the name, dosage and how long the client has taken it. Include prescription and non-prescription medication.

Hearing and vision

Note any difficulties with sight or hearing, particular details of hearing aids, or whether the client needs to wear glasses.

Other agencies

- ○ Name, address and telephone number of general practitioner
- ○ Details of other professionals in regular contact with the client.

Summary of adult case history

Identification details

- ○ Name
- ○ Address
- ○ Telephone number
- ○ Date of birth and age
- ○ Client's identification number

Administrative details

- ○ Date of the interview
- ○ Place of interview
- ○ Name and designation of interviewer.

Referral information

- ○ Name and designation of referring agent
- ○ Reason for the referral/admission
- ○ Date of the referral.

Nature of the problem

- ○ History of the problem
- ○ Effect on Client
- ○ Client's Attitude to the Problem
- ○ Previous History of Assessment
- ○ Previous History of Treatment
- ○ Social History: Family History
- ○ Personal History
- ○ Employment History
- ○ Habits
- ○ Medical History
- ○ Current Health Status
- ○ Hearing and Vision
- ○ Other Agencies.

Paediatric case history

Identification details

- ○ Name
- ○ Address
- ○ Telephone number
- ○ Date of birth and age
- ○ Child's identification number.
- ○ Name by which child is usually known
- ○ Name and address of next of kin/guardians.

Administrative details

- ○ Date of the interview
- ○ Place of the interview
- ○ Name and designation of the interviewer
- ○ Name and address of person attending the interview.

Referral information

- ○ Name and designation of the referring agent
- ○ Reason for the referral
- ○ Date of the referral.

Nature of the problem

- ○ A description of the symptoms
- ○ Date when the problem first started
- ○ The way in which it first became apparent, and who noticed it first.

Record a description of the problem using the parent's/guardian's/child's words.

History of the problem
DEVELOPMENT OF THE PROBLEM
Establish whether the problem has changed in character or severity. Note any circumstances that are associated with these changes.

CONSISTENCY OF THE PROBLEM

Note any times when the problem is better or worse; and any conditions associated with these periods.

Write a clear record of the development of the problem in chronological order. The onset and sequence of symptoms need to be dated as accurately as possible.

Effect on the child and family

Note how the problem is affecting the child and the family. (Relationships; socially; educationally; as well as physical effects.)

Attitude of the child and family to the problem

This section deals with information on the feelings and attitude of the child and family towards the problem, and about the referral itself.

Previous history of assessment

This section refers to previous investigations of the current problem. Find out where the child was seen before, and the name of the professional who dealt with the case. Information about the results of these investigations needs to be obtained.

Previous history of treatment

This section refers to details of previous treatment relevant to the current problem.

- Find out the place of treatment and the name of the clinician
- Note information about the type, length and purpose of the previous treatment
- Establish whether the child is currently receiving treatment elsewhere
- Reasons for a second referral need to be investigated and recorded.

Social history

- *Parents* – Names, ages and occupation of both parents. Find out who lives with the child, and their relationship to the child.

Establish degree of contact between any absent parent and the child.

- ○ *Siblings* – Note the names, ages and their position in the family. Include details of education.
- ○ *Family health* – What is the general health of family members? Is there any family history of illness or disability?
- ○ *Living conditions* – note any special circumstances.

Birth and pregnancy

- ○ Mother's health during pregnancy.
- ○ Date and place of birth; type of delivery; birth weight.
- ○ Note any complications during or immediately after the delivery for mother or baby.
- ○ Length of stay in hospital.
- ○ Health of baby in first few days. Note any admission to special care baby unit (SCBU) with the reason and length of stay.

Medical history

- ○ Periods of hospitalisation with the place, dates and reason for admission
- ○ Details of surgical procedures. (The place where they were performed and the outcome.)
- ○ Major illness or accidents
- ○ Childhood illnesses
- ○ Record of vaccinations.

Record major events in chronological order with the details of the date, circumstances and outcome of each episode.

Feeding and dentition

- ○ Description of feeding history with relevant dates.
- ○ Note any difficulties in feeding or swallowing during infancy.
- ○ Time of teething. Dental history.

Developmental history
Dates that major developmental milestones were achieved in the following areas:

> Gross motor; fine motor; self help skills; toileting; social behaviour; play; and speech and language.

Growth and weight
Note any abnormal trends.

Habits
Eating and sleeping patterns.

Current health status
- ○ Child's current health status.
- ○ *Medication* – Record the name, dosage and how long the child has taken it. Include prescription and non-prescription medication.

Hearing and vision
- ○ Dates of tests with results. Specific details need to be recorded of any hearing or visual problems.
- ○ Names of relevant professionals.

Education
Place of education. Date and age that child started education. Name of head teacher and class teacher. Effects of problem on education.

Other Agencies
- ○ Name, address and telephone number of general practitioner
- ○ Details of other professionals in regular contact with the child.

Summary of Paediatric Case History

Identification details
- ○ Name
- ○ Address
- ○ Telephone number
- ○ Date of birth and age
- ○ Child's identification number.

Administrative details
- ○ Date of the interview
- ○ Place of interview
- ○ Name and designation of interviewer
- ○ Name and address of person attending the interview.

Referral information
- ○ Name and designation of referring agent
- ○ Reason for the referral
- ○ Date of the referral.

Nature of the problem

History of the problem

Effect on the child and family

Attitude of the child and family to the problem

Previous history of assessment

Previous history of treatment

Social history

Birth and pregnancy

Medical history

Feeding and dentition

Developmental history

Growth and weight

Habits

Current health status

Hearing and vision

Education

Other agencies

Giving information

Information provides the client with some control over their situation. An informed client is also a less anxious and therefore a less distressed individual (Wilson-Barnett 1991). Better understanding has also been found to increase satisfaction with clinical interviews (Ley 1982).

What does the client want to know?

The first stage in giving information is to find out what the client wants to know. Do they have any particular worries or concerns? Usually the client wants to know what the problem is, what can be done about it, and when it will go away. In more technical terms they need to know the diagnosis, treatment and prognosis. They may also wonder 'why me' or 'why now'. Even if these questions are not explicitly expressed by the client, they can be used as a guide to the type of information you need to provide.

The most fundamental piece of information required by the client is confirmation of what is causing their problems (although some clients may not, if they fear the worst). Before giving the diagnosis it is useful to say what is functioning normally. The client needs to know the results of all tests, even if no abnormalities were discovered. It also helps to orientate the client if results can be placed within a framework, so that comments are related to normative values. For example, 'Most people pass about two to three pints of urine a day. As you know you are passing more than three times this amount'.

Information provided to clients needs to be accurate. Students on practical placement must consolidate their understanding of relevant topics, and practise explanations on peers, before attempting to explain anything to clients.

The other major question the client will want answered is – 'When will I get better?'. Providing information on the prognosis is a much harder task. It is not always easy to predict the outcome of an illness or the length of recovery. In cases where the news is not good, it is essential that a team approach is used. It is usually better if one member of staff is elected to break the news, although everybody must be aware of what the client has been told, and the response of the client to this news.

Maguire (1991) suggests starting the process by checking the client's awareness of their condition. What do they suspect? The clinician is then able to build on these beliefs and concerns by either confirming or denying them. Sometimes the client will be completely unaware. The client will need time to assimilate the information and its implications. The clinician needs to recognise this period of adjustment, and be prepared for more questions at a later date.

Professionals differ in opinion on whether it is the right of the client to know the full facts about their prognosis. Some feel it is not in the client's best interests to burden them with a poor prognosis. This is an issue that individuals have to work out partly for themselves, and partly within the context of their working environment. The decision should never rest with one individual, but be part of a team decision.

In some instances further investigations are needed. If this is the case, make this clear to the client. But be careful not to raise any false expectations.

Improving memory and understanding of information
Regardless of the content of your message, your aim is to make sure that the client has understood the information and will remember the details. A clear, simple message is much more likely to be remembered. Think of the short, catchy phrases used in adverts. You tend to remember them even if you dislike the message and the product. To simplify your message concentrate on the main points and remove any extraneous details.

Once you have the essence of your message, you can think about how you will structure its delivery. The client is more likely to recall information presented in a logical and ordered fashion. Ley *et al.* (1976) suggest the use of explicit categorisation as a technique. The clinician tells the client what categories of information will be provided. These might include telling the client what is wrong, describing investigations and explaining treatment. The clinician then presents the information category by category. For example, 'First I will tell you what I think is wrong with you'.

How you phrase the message is another consideration. The art of communicating with the client is to have the creativity to express ideas and concepts in language they will understand. One way is to use similar vocabulary and expressions to the client, although this strategy needs to be used with care. Each of us has a dialect and accent, and the use of an uncharacteristic word or phrase will be noticeable to the listener. It is easy to appear condescending or even sarcastic if we mimic other people's words.

A better way is to use your knowledge of the person's interests and background to determine your choice of words; for example, choosing a more technical description of drug therapy for someone who works in the pharmaceutical industry. Again as with any other approach, you need to avoid making assumptions about the level of the client's knowledge, and their ability to assimilate information.

On the whole it is better to avoid using unnecessary medical terminology. Labels do not add to the client's knowledge. They are another barrier to their understanding. It is useful if you think of these terms as name plaques on a series of closed doors. Unless the door is opened, there is no way of knowing what is in the room. If you do need to use a specific term, provide a brief explanation.

Giving information requires flexibility. If your first attempts are unsuccessful, try a different strategy. It is useless to just keep repeating the same message if the client fails to understand. Remember it is difficult for clients to visualise internal organs and how they work, so make use of diagrams and models to help your verbal explanations, or try the use of a simple analogy.

Check that the client's use of a term is the same as yours. Even though you may use the same terms as the client, you may not share the same meaning. What do they mean when say their child is hyperactive? This is a recognised condition with identifiable characteristics. However, the client may be using it to describe a particularly boisterous child whom they are having difficulty in managing.

Giving advice

Part of the information you need to give will be straightforward advice. The type of information you give to the client will be influenced by his attitude and expectations of health care. Does he expect to be cared for or to be able to care for himself? This may mean the difference between a prescribed course of treatment and a negotiated one.

Avoid being too didactic in your approach. Encourage contributions from the client by asking him about how he is coping with the problem. An obese client may say he is cutting down on sweets and cakes. You can follow this up with your advice.

The use of specific rather than general statements have been found to be more effective when giving advice. Avoid vague suggestions like 'You need more exercise'. Your advice will be easier to follow if it states what, when and how. For example, 'Take a twenty minute walk at least three times a week. This will improve your fitness and help in your weight loss programme.' Alternatively, you may want to offer the client a series of choices. These must be real and feasible alternatives. Do not rely on your skills of persuasion to direct the client towards the right choice as you see it.

How much information?

Clients vary in the amount and type of information they require. As their clinician, you need to discover what they want to know as well as what you feel they need to know. You then have to judge the appropriate quantity of information. If you overload the client, he will have difficulty remembering all the details. On the other hand insufficient facts may create dissatisfaction and a lack of understanding. This in turn may lead to failure to comply with treatments.

Dealing with difficult situations in the clinical interview

Most difficult situations in the clinical interview are related to the emotional reactions of the client. The most common feeling is distress. But health professionals also are increasingly having to deal with angry and aggressive clients. Here are some guidelines for dealing with these types of client:

Dealing with the distressed client

Although clients vary in their reactions, distress and anxiety are common. Sometimes the client may become openly emotional. Fear of having to deal with these situations leads some interviewers to suppress this side of the interview. They carefully avoid any reference to the client's feelings. Any distress on the part of the client is disregarded or brushed over.

This type of attitude is not conducive to establishing a good relationship with the client. They will feel ignored, angry or embarrassed by the apparent lack of concern. The clinician needs to offer support and reassurance by acknowledging the client's feelings. This might be verbally, for example 'I realise this has been a terrible shock for you'. It may be through touch, a hand on the client's shoulder, or the tone of voice you use. You may also need to explore the source of the client's anxiety, and offer advice or information if appropriate.

Dealing with the angry client

Occasionally the health professional is confronted by an angry client. A variety of different events may have triggered their anger. It may even be part of their health problem, for instance in mental illness.

It is better if anger is dealt with early on before it has a chance to intensify. Look out for any signs in the client's behaviour that may indicate she is becoming angry. This may be in her body language, tone or volume of voice or in how she phrases a question.

Your first response will be to listen to the client. This is critical. Never try to rationalise or allow yourself to get angry. Show the client that you are listening by using non-verbal and paralinguistic behaviours. However, avoid using too much eye-contact as this may be perceived as threatening or intimidating.

Once you have given the client a chance to let off steam, you need to acknowledge her anger (Maguire 1991). This shows that you are aware of how she is feeling. If appropriate, ask questions to help her express the source of her anger. These should be genuine enquiries. Let her know if you already know what she is angry about.

Try to resolve any issues with the client. Ideally you will be able to offer a solution to the client. This may be as simple as allowing her the opportunity to talk through her feelings. Sometimes an explanation needs to be provided. Avoid becoming defensive. For example, trying to counter a complaint from a client by saying she has failed to attend appointments. Use a calm and direct manner when explaining to the client.

Some clients may wish to lodge a formal complaint. It is important for your own protection that you follow the guidelines laid down by your employers. Check your procedures carefully.

Dealing with the aggressive client

Sometimes the angry client becomes the aggressive client. In dealing with this type of individual, you need to ensure your safety and the safety of other clients.

Make sure you are not alone with the person. Ask another member of staff to be with you, when seeing the person. Avoid arranging appointments in isolated locations. This would include the client's home or during an evening clinic when there are few staff around.

Regardless of where you see the client, you need to ensure that you can summon help quickly. Carry a personal alarm at all times. You also need to familiarise yourself with how to contact security, and the use of any security systems like panic buttons.

If a client suddenly becomes angry, you may need to remove yourself and other clients from the situation. Leave the area until help has arrived.

As a general safety rule it is a good idea if you get into the habit of informing other staff of your whereabouts. If you go on a home visit, make sure somebody knows where you are and when you are expected back.

These are general guidelines only. If you work regularly with aggressive clients, you need additional training.

Dealing with clients who have a communication difficulty

Communication difficulties are associated with a number of medical conditions. These may result in a variety of speech, language and communication problems of varying degrees of severity. However, these difficulties do not automatically mean that the client has any cognitive problems.

Difficulties may not always be apparent at first. The following questions will help you identify clients who may have communication difficulties:

- Does the client have difficulty in understanding instructions?
- Do they seem to be struggling to follow conversation?
- Do they seem to forget words?
- Do they have difficulty in expressing themselves?
- Are their sentences disjointed or odd in any way?
- Is their speech slurred or unclear?
- Do they seem to be responding or acting inappropriately?

If you suspect that a client has a communication difficulty you can get advice from a speech and language therapist.

Remember the client with a communication difficulty is likely to feel isolated, lonely and confused. This may turn into anger and frustration at staff. Use these guidelines to ease communication during the interview.

General guidelines

- Looking and listening are important. Does the client have a hearing aid or glasses? Encourage the client to wear their hearing aid. The hearing aid department who issued the aid will be able to assist you if there are any problems. These departments are usually based in a hospital. Glasses need to be clean and appropriate for the task. For instance, does the client need different glasses for reading?

- Reduce distractions by taking the client to a quiet area where there will be no interruptions. The client will find it difficult to concentrate with a radio or television on in the background.

- Remember clients with communication difficulties quickly tire. Keep your interview as brief as possible.

- Be patient. Some clients may take longer to respond. Give them the feeling that you have all the time in the world, even if you are rushed off your feet. Any efforts to hurry the client will usually hinder their communication.

- Encourage the client to communicate. Show him you are interested in finding out his views.

- Face the client, and encourage him to look at you.

You may have difficulty in understanding the speech of some clients. Here are some strategies for helping both you and the client:

- Tell the client if you have not understood something he has said. Encourage him to repeat words or say things in a different way or use writing or drawing.

- Repeat back to the client what you think he has said. This will help you check your understanding.

- Ask the client to slow down if he is speaking too fast.

- You may need to give the client a rest and try again later.

Some clients may have difficulty in understanding what you are saying. Use the following strategies to aid their comprehension:

- Make sure you have the client's attention before you say anything.

- Talk slowly and clearly using short sentences. But avoid talking down to the client.

- Check if their yes/no response is reliable. (Use simple questions to which you *know* the answer – Is it raining outside? Are you married?)
- If necessary use alternative means to help the client to understand – pictures, gestures, pointing. Remember a few clients may have difficulties in even understanding these things.
- Try to cue the client using forced alternatives like 'Do you want tea or coffee?'

The client with a hearing loss

About one in six people have some sort of hearing loss. Many of these will be elderly, because the incidence of hearing loss increases with age. Some will wear hearing aids, which improve hearing by making sounds louder. However, hearing aids do not restore hearing to normal. Sound is still distorted and difficult for the person to understand.

This is why many people also depend on lip reading, a technique that relies on recognising words by the movements of the lips and tongue. This is not always easy as many sounds look the same. (You can demonstrate this for yourself. Watch in a mirror as you mouth the words pan, man and ban.) Because of these difficulties lip readers rely on other cues from the context, the rhythm of speech and the facial expression of the speaker.

Clients who present with a hearing loss have special needs in terms of communication. Here are some guidelines on meeting these requirements.

Be alert for clients with a hearing loss

Be alert for any signs that may indicate a hearing loss in the client. Does the client appear confused? Irritated? Embarrassed? Blank? Do you have to repeat words or sentences? Are responses to questions inappropriate? Do they speak with an unusually loud or quiet voice? Look out for other clues like how loud the client has the television or radio.

Create a sympathetic listening environment

Hearing aids tend to amplify background noise. The sound of chairs scraping, footsteps, or plates and cutlery being placed on tables are exaggerated. This makes it difficult to distinguish the much softer sounds of speech.

Try to talk to your client in a quiet area. A side room is better than the middle of the ward, and an office is better than a corridor. A room with carpets and curtains is ideal as the soft furnishings help to damp down extraneous noises.

Help the person to understand your speech

(1) Make sure the client can see your face, especially your mouth. When you are talking:

- Avoid covering your mouth with your hand.

- Remember that looking down at your notes or glancing away will obscure the view of your face.

- Keep your face on the same level as the client's. This applies particularly to children, but also to those clients who are lying down or in a wheel chair. Try to seat yourself at the same height.

- Avoid standing with your back to the window as your face will be in shadow. A well-lit room is better for lip reading.

- Stand or sit between 3 feet (90cm) and 6 feet (1.8m) away from the client. This is the ideal distance for people to lip read and hear your voice through their hearing aid.

(2) Tell the person the topic or subject matter before you start talking about it. This helps them to tune into the conversation much quicker.

(3) Speak clearly with a slightly raised voice. Avoid shouting or exaggerating your articulation as this will distort your lip patterns.

(4) The lip reader will be following whole phrases rather than word by word or sound by sound. So avoid breaking up your message into one or two words like 'Your' 'operation' 'is tomorrow'. Keep to the natural phrasing groups of the sentence 'Your operation is tomorrow'.

(5) If there are several people involved in the interview, agree to take turns at speaking. The client can only lip read one person at a time.

(6) Check that the person is following what you are saying. Do not rely on head nods, or yes and no responses as an indication the person has understood. Ask questions or get the person to summarise. Repeat sentences again if necessary, and then rephrase if the person is still having difficulty.

(7) The person will be unable to lip read you and look at any visual material like leaflets, diagrams or models. Allow the person some time to look at the material, and then get their attention before talking again.

Help to prevent isolation and fear

Keep the client informed about what is happening to them, using a variety of communication modes. These include writing, drawing and non-verbal communication like facial expression. Clients who are signers need interpreting services. See the section on 'Working with Interpreters' for more details.

Making notes

Health professionals are required by law to record in writing any contact with clients. In an initial interview you will need to take a thorough and comprehensive case history. You may want to discuss with the client who will have access to this information. This should certainly be the case if students are taking any notes.

Note taking is difficult if you are trying to maintain a conversation with the client. The skill of the effective interviewer is the ability to attend to the client as well as recording all the relevant information. This means looking at the client when they are responding, rather than immediately recording their responses. You need to develop the ability to quickly note the salient points of the discussion. Otherwise there will be lengthy pauses in between questions as you write up your notes.

Closing the interview

The closure of the interview will include a summary of the main points of your discussion, and a final check with the client that all areas have been covered. You may also want to give the person an opportunity to add any other information.

The final point is the proposed course of action for the client. This will cover any follow-up that is necessary, including referral to other agencies and details of treatment.

Action Points

Try these activities with a friend or colleague.

(1) Discuss with a partner when you have had difficulties attending to a client. Use Burnard's description of attention domains (see p.91) as a basis for your discussion.

(2) Listen to a partner tell you about a problem they are trying to deal with like noisy neighbours or tax problems. Concentrate on listening to them without allowing your thoughts to interfere. Reverse the situation so that your partner is listening to you. Afterwards discuss how it felt to listen and to be listened to in this focused way.

(3) Interview a partner about a special event in their past. Your partner should aim to be rather vague and forgetful. Can you improve the accuracy of their information giving?

(4) Practise explaining a medical condition or a treatment approach to a friend with a non-medical background. How much can they repeat back to you? How accurate is it? Do they agree with you on which points were the most important?

(5) Role play a clinical interview with your partner. Record the interview using a camcorder or tape recorder. Play back the interview and discuss the following questions with your partner.

- How did you start the interview?

- Did the interviewee have an opportunity to express the problem in their own words? At what point did this happen in the interview?

Analyse each question.

- What type of question was it?
- What sort of response did it elicit?
- Could you have phrased it better? If so, how?
- What behaviours on your part encouraged a greater contribution from the client?
- Did you give any information?
- What pieces of information did you choose to give?
- Were these in response to a request by the interviewee?
- How did you structure your information giving?

Summary Points

- The clinical interview is your main point of contact with the client. It will form a major part of your diagnostic and therapeutic procedures. It is also crucial in helping you to establish and maintain a relationship with your client.

- Pre-interview preparation will involve you in gathering information about the client's previous medical history, his present condition and the reasons for the referral.

- Your preparation will also include making sure that the environment is conducive to communication. (The arrangement of the waiting area and the clinic room can affect how much clients contribute to the interview.)

- Your need to establish a rapport with the client from the start of the interview. It will encourage his confidence and trust in you as a professional.

- One of your primary aims in a clinical interview is to gather information that will assist you in making a diagnosis and establishing the needs of the client in terms of therapy or treatment.

- There are numerous strategies you can use to make sure this information is relevant, accurate and as complete as possible. These include asking for examples, using clarification questions and offering suggestions.

- Information giving is also an important part of the clinical interview. Providing the client with information reduces anxiety and distress. Better understanding has also been found to increase client satisfaction.

Interviewing Skills in Context
Appraisal Interviews

In recent years the health service has seen the introduction of a system of appraisal, sometimes referred to as individual performance review (IPR). A system of appraisal is familiar to management in industry but is a relatively new concept to health care workers. Randall *et al.* (1984, p.12) defined an appraisal system as 'a procedure that helps the collecting, checking, sharing, giving and using of information collected from and about people at work for the purposes of adding to their performance at work'.

What is the purpose of an appraisal system?

As stated by Randall, appraisal is a way of gathering and sharing information between employer and employee. It also has another important role, that of maintaining and improving work performance. For the manager it is an opportunity to learn exactly who is doing what within his department. For the individual it is an opportunity to identify and plan self development through further training or additional responsibilities. Ideally, the whole process is one that encourages the exchange of ideas. Its conclusion is the establishment of mutually agreed targets for the appraisee.

The setting of objectives for individuals makes explicit what is expected of the employee and provides them with feedback on what is valued by their employer. These might be management, service or individual objectives. An objective or goal is a statement about the results to be achieved by the individual (Maddux 1987). They must be achievable, have a fixed time-frame and be supported by the necessary resources. An example of an objective for a speech therapist might be to become skilled in working with clients with dysphagia by completing a post graduate training course within the next year.

How is appraisal conducted?

An appraisal system involves each employee having an identified appraiser. A supervisor or manager with expertise and experience relevant to the appraisee is the ideal choice. The bulk of the appraisal process is carried out during the appraisal interview. This is a meeting between the appraiser and the appraisee.

What is the appraisal process?

There are five main elements in the process of appraisal:

(1) Gathering information

(2) Sharing information

(3) Recognising achievements

(4) Problem solving

(5) Planning.

(1) Information gathering

Both the appraiser and the appraisee need to spend time gathering information for the appraisal interview. This includes information about performance; staff development; and special activities carried out during the period covered by the appraisal. Part of this process may involve the appraisee completing a questionnaire and attending a pre-appraisal meeting. Some organisations have specific guidelines on the sort of information required for the appraisal.

An *appraiser* needs to seek information on the requirements of the post as well as the performance of the post holder. These will come from a variety of sources that include:

- A job analysis
- A work programme
- Previous appraisal objectives
- Reports from supervisors
- Feedback from colleagues
- Feedback from clients
- Specific examples of appraisee's achievements.

The *appraisee* can collate pertinent information such as:

- A description of their main roles and responsibilities

- ○ An estimate of the time they spend on each area of responsibility
- ○ A list of the main objectives for each of these areas
- ○ A record of performance for each of these objectives (i.e. what has been achieved)
- ○ Attendance records of any training received
- ○ Evidence of additional qualifications with the dates obtained.

(*See the action points at the end of this section for more help on preparing information for an appraisal.*)

(2) Sharing information

The appraisal interview is about exchanging information. Both the appraiser and the appraisee need to provide input at this stage. Details need to be confirmed and any ambiguities clarified. This is an opportunity for both the appraiser and the appraisee to correct any misinformation.

(3) Recognising achievements

An appraisal interview is incomplete if the achievements of the employee pass unnoticed. Apart from the mutual satisfaction of recognising a job well done, the organisation also benefits from the increase in motivation that is a likely result of this verbal reward. It confirms to the appraisee exactly what their employer values.

(4) Problem solving

It may be necessary to take a problem solving approach if there is a difference between expectations and the results. Both the appraiser and the appraisee will be involved in identifying problems and offering solutions.

(5) Planning

The final part of the appraisal is to agree a set of objectives and draw up a plan of how these will be achieved. Objectives need to be placed within a time-frame, which is usually based around the period of the appraisal system. In some cases it may be necessary to have a shorter or longer period of review. A series of subgoals can be used for a long term project. For example, the goal of implementing a computerised system for recording client data may need several subgoals. These might include devising databases, implementing training, and supervising staff in their initial use of the computers. The action plan needs to detail any training or allocation of specific resources that are required in order for the individual to meet the objectives.

What is the role of the appraiser?

Preparation

Appraisal is about communication. So it is important that you make sure the appraisee knows what will happen and when. He will need to understand the appraisal system, before he is able to appreciate its purpose and value. In-service training is one way of introducing staff to the system.

The appraisee also needs to be aware of the time-table of events. For example, you will have a set period in which to complete your interviews, so let your appraisee know the time-frame in which you are working. Agree a mutually convenient date and time for the appraisal interview, that gives both you and the appraisee enough time to prepare.

Your interview needs to be carefully structured. A lack of structure will result in the interview becoming rambling and purposeless. An inappropriate or rigid structure may prevent a proper exchange of ideas. Think about your general aims for the interview. These might include:

- consolidating information
- gathering new information
- giving feedback
- resolving problems
- agreeing a set of objectives
- agreeing an action plan.

Within these general aims identify specific aims that relate to the appraisee. These might be to give praise for a successful initiative, to identify objectives for implementing newly learnt skills or to discuss the failure to satisfy previous objectives. Estimate roughly how much time you will need to accomplish each aim.

You now have a plan for your interview, but do not treat this as a definitive blueprint. Your aims will be modified once you have met with the appraisee and information has been shared and exchanged.

Setting the scene

It is important that the appraisee feels you are ready, willing, and able to listen and respond to their needs. Arrange your diary so that you start punctually, and there is adequate time to complete the interview. Remember your appraisee will have a busy schedule too. He will not want to be kept waiting.

The choice of venue for your interview is also important. Make sure you have a comfortable room that offers privacy and is free from interruptions. Arrange the seating in an informal way.

Opening statements

As the appraiser you will generally take the lead by initiating the discussion with some welcoming comments. Remind the appraisee of the purpose of the interview and re-iterate the ground rules. It is essential at this early stage to agree on the aims of the meeting (Hunt 1992), otherwise you will be talking at cross-purposes. This is also your opportunity to emphasise the co-operative and dynamic nature of the appraisal.

Eliciting information from the appraisee

You will have formed ideas about possible objectives from the information you gathered before the interview. However, these are to be viewed as tentative ideas that will form the basis of your discussion, and are not a ready made prescription to be imposed on the appraisee.

One of the purposes of the interview is to expand on this information base. There are a number of different ways of going about it. Maddux (1987) suggests starting the discussion on a positive note by inviting the appraisee to talk about their achievements.

An alternative approach is to deal with each area of responsibility at a time. Otherwise the appraisee may have difficulty concentrating on achievements if they are worried about possible criticisms (Croner 1985). The way that you approach the interview is really a matter of individual choice. Whatever you decide, tell the appraisee how you are going to structure the interview.

Encouraging the appraisee

The use of an open style of question like 'Tell me about...' will get the appraisee talking. Using pauses is also a powerful way of encouraging contributions from the appraisee. Leave a gap after the appraisee makes a comment and he will probably add some more information. The aim is for the majority of the speaking time to be used by the appraisee.

Recognising achievements

It is important to praise successes and recognise how these have been brought about. Often people are reluctant to 'blow their own trumpet', and you may have to give a few examples of their achievements to get them started. This discussion can then broaden out to other issues. The aim is to confirm and add to your knowledge of the appraisee and their job.

Problem solving

Try to elicit what the problems are from the appraisee. You are more likely to achieve their co-operation if they have some awareness of their difficulties. Acknowledging their ability to evaluate their performance will encourage them to discuss difficulties, for example, 'Yes, that comment shows a lot of insight.'

Sometimes it will be necessary for you to highlight problem areas. Always start by re-stating the objective or standard that has not been met. Then ask the appraisee for reasons. For example, 'The waiting list for first appoint-ments seems to be extended beyond our four week limit, which is one of the indicators for our quality assurance. Why do you feel this is happening?' Always specify the problem with examples. Nothing will be achieved by labelling the person as incompetent or lazy. It will only provoke anger or make the appraisee feel inadequate.

Planning

This is a joint process between you and the appraisee. Use open questions to elicit suggestions and ideas. If the appraisee makes a tentative proposal, reinforce these with prompts like 'go on' and 'tell me more'. This is a time to listen. Resist the urge to join in with your own thoughts on the subject, until the appraisee has finished.

Completing the interview

The way that you complete your interview will significantly effect its outcome (Koontz and O'Donnell 1984). When planning your appraisal, allow time at the end to give a summary of your discussion. This will include a statement of the agreed objectives, the time-frame for achieving these objectives and the necessary resources to implement them. Alternatively, ask the appraisee to summarise.

This is the last opportunity for the appraisee to respond and to correct any misrepresentations. So ask the appraisee if they have any further questions or comments to make.

Draw up an action plan based on your summary. It is essential to keep a written copy of this plan, which must be agreed and signed by both parties.

What is the role of the appraisee?

Preparation

Preparation is vital. You need to allocate time and effort to the process. It may seem a tedious and time-consuming business, but appraisal affects your everyday work throughout the year. It is useful to think of the appraisal as an on-going process, not just a once yearly event. You are working on your agreed objectives throughout the year. The appraisal is a way of reflecting this effort and commitment to the job.

There are three main things you need to communicate in the interview:

○ A realistic evaluation of your work performance

○ Proposals for dealing with any unfulfilled objectives

○ Ideas for new objectives.

Use the action points at the end of the section to help you plan your appraisal.

Selling yourself

It is easy to focus on problems and forget achievements. Remember to talk about your successes. State these clearly, and avoid the temptation to waffle. This often happens if we feel embarrassed. We are afraid of appearing big-headed if we talk about ourselves directly. This is more often the case with women than men. Women are traditionally less competitive, and have less experience of putting themselves forward. If you have done the hard work, you deserve the credit.

Dealing with criticism

It may be the case that you have failed to fulfil an objective or the appraiser has other specific criticisms. You are on much stronger ground when you are able to identify these problems yourself. It is important to raise any obstacles to your fulfilling your objectives with your manager as soon as possible. Do not store up difficulties for the appraisal interview.

However, there will be occasions where you will need to respond to criticism within the appraisal. Dickson (1982) suggests responding to valid criticism with what she has termed negative assertion. This is basically agreeing with the criticism and accepting its validity. For example, 'Yes, you're right. The waiting lists are behind.' Avoid the urge to get defensive or put yourself down (Butler 1992). This allows the discussion to move on to improving the situation.

Criticism that you feel is unjust needs to be dealt with in a different way. It is often the case with unfair criticism that it comes at you completely out of the blue. As you have had no time to prepare a response, take your time before replying. Ask for concrete examples. You also have the right to know who has made a specific criticism. Dispute any comments you feel are unjustified. Phrases like 'That's untrue' or 'I can't accept that' expressed in a definite manner will make your message clear (Dickson 1982).

Suggesting a proposal

The appraisal is an opportunity for you to put forward ideas and suggestions. Do not miss out on this chance to influence your work pattern. Know what you want to say. You are more likely to persuade your manager if you have specific targets in mind. Instead of saying 'I would like to do more training', give examples such as 'I am interested in setting up in-service training on counselling the bereaved'. Be ready to support your proposal with reasons, although Hunt (1992) warns against diluting your argument with too many justifications.

Planning

You have an equal share in planning goals. Make this an active role. Check out what you are being asked to do. Listen to the appraiser carefully. Are the objectives realistic and appropriate? Is the time-frame sensible? Do you have the necessary support to fulfil the objectives? Never accept an objective if you are unhappy with it. Make it clear what your objections are and try to negotiate a more agreeable alternative.

Why do appraisals go wrong?

There are a number of reasons why appraisal systems do not work either for the benefit of the individual or the organisation. A less than satisfactory appraisal for the employee will eventually have an impact on the efficiency of the service. Therefore it is important to sort out problems.

Difficulties can arise in the communication between appraiser and appraisee, or at a higher level in the organisation. Do you recognise any of the following from your experience of appraisal systems?

Problems at an organisational level

- The system is ill defined
- The system is not equally applied to all staff
- Staff receive no or inadequate training
- Staff do not understand the system

  ◦ Staff do not appreciate the benefits of the system to them as individuals.

Problems at an individual level

  ◦ Inadequate preparation
  ◦ Failure to understand the nature and purpose of the interview
  ◦ The style and tone of the interview prevents a two-way communication of ideas
  ◦ The interview lacks structure
  ◦ Confidentiality is breached.

Improving communication will solve many of these problems. If you are in the process of reviewing your system follow these guidelines:

✧ **Communicate information about the system through regular in-service training for all staff.**

✧ **Provide staff manuals that detail the appraisal system including procedures and the responsibilities of individuals.**

✧ **Give appraisers training in interviewing skills.**

✧ **Encourage appraisers to regularly review their skills. Provide opportunities for newly appointed appraisers to meet with more experienced colleagues.**

✧ **Publish the time-table for the appraisal process.**

Action Points

Appraiser

Use the checklist below to evaluate the effectiveness of your interviewing skills. Complete this by yourself or set up a role-play situation with colleagues.

☐ Did you state the purpose of the interview?

☐ Did you discuss the format the interview would take?

☐ Did you establish and show recognition for the appraisee's achievements?

☐ Was there a balance between open and closed questions?

☐ Did you avoid leading questions or statements?

☐ Did you use verbal and non-verbal means to encourage contributions from the appraisee?

☐ Did you make it clear what expectations you had of the appraisee?

☐ Did you support your criticisms with specific examples?

☐ Did you acknowledge when the appraisee identified a problem?

☐ Did you provide a summary at the end?

☐ Was the appraisee asked whether he had any more questions?

☐ Were the objectives clearly stated with an appropriate time-scale?

☐ What proportion of the time did you spend listening?

☐ What proportion of the time did you spend talking?

Make a note of things you said or did. This might be a particular question or the use of a non-verbal signal like nodding. Next to it note how you think it affected the interviewee. For example:

Appraiser	*Appraisee*
Nodding and saying 'Go on'	Talked more
Frowning	Hesitated

Appraisees

Thorough preparation before your appraisal, although a chore, is essential. You need to:

- Know your own strengths and weaknesses
- Understand your work patterns

- Evaluate your work performance
- Consider how problems may be resolved
- Plan your career.

Use these exercises to help your preparation.

(1) Think about your strengths and weaknesses. List these under the following headings:

- Personal qualities (for example, personality, attitude, motivation)
- Skills
- Experience
- Qualifications.

(2) List the main areas of your work.

For example:

- Clinical (e.g. treating clients, liaison with other professionals)
- Supervising staff
- Management (e.g. planning budgets)
- Administration (e.g. compiling statistics, filing, arranging appointments)
- Teaching or training others
- Receiving training
- Research
- Professional activities (e.g. attending conferences or meetings of your professional body).

Prioritise these areas according to your main responsibilities. Make a list starting with the area that you feel is the most important.

(3) Think about the amount of time you spend on each area. You may want to look at your work pattern over one week, a month, a school term or during one shift. This will depend on your individual work load. Choose a period of time that will reflect the overall pattern of work within the appraisal period.

In most organisations this is a year. So if each week in the year is the same, use your weekly activities to calculate your work pattern. If your work varies throughout a school term, but each term's work within a year is similar, use this as the measurement. In some cases the work may be so varied that patterns within the whole year will need to be examined. Try to work out the actual hours and the percentage of the whole. For example a weekly pattern might look something like this:

	Hours	%
Clinical	28	70
Supervising staff	6	15
Administration	4	10
Receiving training	2	5

Plot your work areas onto a pie chart. This will give you an immediate visual impression of how you spend your time. Compare your chart with your priority list. How much time is spent on your priority area? Do you spend a little bit of time on each area? Do some areas always have a large chunk of your time?

You will now have a much clearer understanding of your work pattern.

(4) Write down your objectives for each of your work areas, with details of the time-frame and the resources. Use your previous appraisal objectives. (If this is your first appraisal think about what your personal goals have been in these areas.) Make a separate list for those objectives you have achieved. Add any other achievements not directly related to specific objectives.

Use the table 2.1 for those objectives that you did not fulfil. Write down the reason or reasons you feel they were not achieved. These might be personal such as poor planning or time-management, or the problem might lie at an organisational level, for example a lack of resources. You might have found that in attempting to fulfil the objectives that they were inappropriate or unrealistic. Next, write down what would help you to achieve your objectives. The table contains several ideas for solutions including further training, experience and resources. Use the last two columns for any other ideas.

Table 2.1 Self-evaluation of appraisal objectives

Objective	Reason for non-achievement	Experience	Training	Resources		

(5) Think about what your new objectives might be.

Ask yourself the following questions:

How do you feel about your work?

- ☐ Bored
- ☐ Frustrated
- ☐ Challenged
- ☐ Out of your depth
- ☐ Stimulated
- ☐ Interested
- ☐ Satisfied
- ☐ Irritated

Do you want to try new areas?

What do you like about your job?

What do you dislike about your job?

Are your talents being used?

Your responses will give you ideas on changes to make to your work responsibilities. Plan to increase the positive aspects of your work, and reduce the negative ones.

Your objectives need to reflect your overall career plan. Know where you are going and why. View each objective as a step nearer your goal.

Summary Points

- An appraisal system is a way of sharing information between the employee and the employer.

- The purpose of appraisal is to maintain and improve work performance by setting specific objectives.

- Each employee has an identified appraiser. The core of the appraisal is the interview between the appraiser and the appraisee.

- There are five main elements to the appraisal process. These are:
  - Gathering information
  - Sharing of information
  - Recognising achievements
  - Problem solving
  - Planning.

- The appraisal interview is a two-way process. Both the appraiser and the appraisee have a joint responsibility to evaluate work performance and plan appropriate objectives.

- The completion of the appraisal will result in an action plan for the appraisee. This will comprise a statement of the agreed objectives, the time-frame for achieving these objectives and the necessary resources to implement them.

- A poor appraisal will affect the efficiency of an organisation. Improving communication helps to avoid some of the reasons for appraisals not working. This includes regular training and information for appraisers and appraisees.

Interviewing Skills in Context
Recruitment Interviews

One of the main roles of the manager is recruiting suitable staff for vacant posts. This is achieved by advertising, shortlisting applications and inviting suitable candidates to interview. This section offers some practical advice on the recruitment process for both the manager and the candidate. Although the information is divided into two sections – 'Recruiting The Candidate' and 'Applying for a Post', the reader is strongly advised to read both. In this way they will gain an insight into each side of the process.

Recruiting the candidate

Recruitment interviews differ significantly from other types of interview in their structure and the roles of the participants. Traditionally the focus of the interviewer has been on establishing and consolidating information about the candidate. There has also been the more personal factor of finding out if they liked them as a person. On the basis of this information the interviewer decided on the suitability of the candidate for the post. The emphasis has always been firmly on the interviewer making the selection.

The power of the candidate to select tends to be overlooked, especially in times of massive unemployment. The assumption is that 'he has applied, he must want the job'. However, like the interviewer, he will also be making judgements about whether to accept the post if offered. This has always occurred, but maybe in a covert fashion. The way that the interview is structured will either inhibit or facilitate this evaluation.

There are advantages to both parties in encouraging the candidate to have an active role in the selection process. You are saved time if unsuitable candidates drop out at an early stage. The candidate is spared the effort of preparing for an interview, if he knows he lacks the basic credentials. There are also long-term benefits. Recruiting is expensive. The aim is to retain staff for as long as they are needed. A quick turn-over of staff is to be avoided. By providing information about the service, you are giving the candidate a more realistic view of the working environment. They do not have to wait till they have started work to find out if they like it.

Interviews are only part of the selection process. The first step in the recruitment process is to identify the sort of candidate you hope to recruit. Before you can start to advertise you need to establish:

- What is the exact nature of the post?
- What sort of person will suit this post?

You need to draw up a job description and a job specification.

Job description

A job description details information about the post. It also describes the type of duties in which the post holder will be expected to engage. It informs the applicant exactly what the post will be like, it will stimulate interest, and encourage unsuitable candidates to de-select themselves. Make your job description as comprehensive as possible.

A job description will include the following information:

- Title of the Post
- Location
- Number of hours
- Grade
- Salary
- Person to whom post holder is responsible (or immediate line manager)
- Person to whom post holder is accountable (head of department or service)
- Job Summary: to include the purpose and scope of the post holders work
- Main tasks and responsibilities: these should be listed with a brief description
- Responsibility of the post holder in evaluating performance.

Here is an example of a job description for a speech and language therapist:

Job description

Post: Specialist Speech and Language Therapist

Location: Child Developmental Centre, St. Brythe's Hospital

Number of hours: 40 hours

Grade: 29–31

Salary: £19,496–£21,072

Responsible to: Principal Speech and Language Therapist

Accountable to: Therapy Manager

Job Summary: The post holder is responsible for the organisation and provision of a specialist clinical service, consisting of assessment, diagnosis and treatment of children referred to the Child Development Centre.

Main duties and responsibilities:

(1) To assess, diagnose and treat communication disorders in children referred to the Child Development Centre.

(2) To participate in the multi-disciplinary management of the child.

(3) To liaise with relevant professionals in the health, education, and social services regarding individual client care.

(4) To contribute to statementing procedures for individual clients as necessary.

(5) To carry out administrative duties as appropriate.

(6) To participate in staff appraisal.

Job Specification

A job specification describes the qualities of the post holder rather than the post itself. Some of these qualities will be essential and others desirable (Pedler *et al.* 1994). The essential qualities will form your shortlisting criteria. Make these clear to the candidate. You might also consider listing any factors that would disqualify a candidate.

Consider the following areas when drawing up your specification:

- Education

- Qualifications
- Training
- Skills
- Experience
- Personal characteristics
- Any other special requirements (e.g., driving licence).

Your advertisement will be based on key information from the job description and job specification. You need to supply the relevant information to your human resources department, who will prepare and place the advertisement.

Candidates who apply for the post need to be sent a copy of the job description and information on the shortlisting criteria. In addition it is useful to send a job information package.

Job information package

A job information package provides candidates with information about the organisation and the department. This will stimulate interest in the post, and give the candidate a feel for the work environment. Here are some ideas of information you could include:

Description of the organisation

This is a description of the overall employing body. It will include the following details:

- The type of organisation (acute services, hospice, medical school, community trust)
- A brief history
- The size of the organisation (numbers of clients; staff; students if it is an educational establishment)
- The area from which the population is drawn
- A brief statement of the philosophy of the organisation
- Recent major developments (Trust status, building renovations).

Description of the department/service

As with the overall organisation, it will be interesting to detail the history, size and structure of your department or service. If your department/service is small, supply a list of staff names and responsibilities. You might also like to include any specific characteristics that would attract a candidate, such as involvement in a research project or a special association.

Information about prospective candidates

Most of the detail about the prospective candidate will be in your job specification. Use this document to expand on the attitudes, values, and disposition that are relevant to the department or service as a whole.

Information about the Selection Process

Let the candidates know when you intend to short list and the dates of the interview. Specify if informal visits are encouraged and provide the name of a contact person. Give details about any special requirements, for example, if candidates have to make a presentation.

Here is an example of a job package:

Specialist health visitor

Tredmore Health Services provides community health care for an inner city population of 337,988 people living in the boroughs of Dore and Trainton. It obtained Trust status in 1991 with the aim of maintaining its comprehensive and high quality service. There are currently 876 people employed by the Trust in a range of professions that include nursing, medical and therapy services.

Greenley Centre has recently been relocated to new, purpose built accommodation. The centre is situated close to the busy Greenley high street with its many shops and restaurants. Parking for staff cars is provided at the rear of the centre.

The successful applicant will complete a team of five full-time health visitors. The main focus of the post will initially be to develop support networks for carers. The post holder will be expected to work closely with the local authority and voluntary organisations.

Applicants are welcome to make an informal visit to the practice. Please contact Dr Briey.

Shortlisted candidates will be invited for interview by 25 November. Interviews will be held on the afternoon of 6 December.

Interviewing a candidate

Use your essential criteria to shortlist candidates. You need to whittle the number down to five or six.

The human resources department usually deal with inviting candidates to interview and requesting references. You might want to specify that the referees comment on particular aspects; for example, amount of sick leave.

Some people prefer to read references before the interview; others prefer to form their impression of the candidate first. It is a matter of personal choice.

Organising the interview

Book a room in a quiet area that is away from distractions, particularly any noise. Arrange for a member of staff to receive the candidates on arrival, and show them to the waiting area (Goodworth 1979). This person can also be enlisted to guard against any interruptions.

Structuring the interview

Most selection interviews are conducted by a panel of interviewers, who are chosen for a variety of reasons. The usual format is to have the manager to whom the post holder is accountable, the first line manager of the post, and a representative from human resources. Occasionally other staff are invited to join the panel. For example, a clinician with special expertise regarding the post, or a representative from another service who will be working closely with the post holder.

The panel needs to decide in advance how they wish to structure the interview. The main decision is the election of a chair, and a discussion of the role this person will play. A chair acts as a focus for the candidate and provides a structure to the interview. They will be the person to draw the interview to a close, checking there are no more questions from either the panel or the candidate.

There are two types of interview – formal and informal. These are distinguished by the lay-out of the room, and the style of interaction with the candidate.

In a formal interview, the candidate is seated opposite the panel members, who are usually situated behind a desk at some distance away. The main emphasis is on information gathering using specific questions. Initiations by the candidate will be minimal.

Many professions favour an informal interview. Chairs are arranged in a semi-circle with the distance between the candidate and the interviewers much smaller than in a formal interview. A small coffee table can be used as an unobtrusive barrier if necessary. Interaction in these interviews is less formal, with the candidate being encouraged to make contributions. Questions are more likely to be of the open type. This is the type of interview you would use for a candidate who has been head hunted.

The members of a panel need to agree on the approach to the interview. A formal style will require each interviewer asking a specific number of questions. A less formal style might opt for a specified amount of time for each interviewer. It is then up to the individual what and how many questions they ask. There is also the issue of consistency in approach to each candidate. Do you repeat the same questions? This is a fair method, but makes for a less individualised approach. Some pertinent points may be overlooked. In some cases it can encourage the interviewer to lose track of the purpose of the interview. I once attended an interview where I was asked a series of questions, which were duly ticked or crossed according to my response. The interviewer barely made eye-contact. A pre-interview questionnaire would have dealt with all the questions. There were so many other interesting questions that could have been asked. Instead of checking whether I had training in a specific teaching programme, why not find out how it had changed my clinical practice or why I thought it was relevant to the post under discussion? Aim to be flexible in your approach.

Preparing questions

The one thing that concerns most novice interviewers is choosing the questions. Your role on the panel will provide some indication of what you need to be asking. If you are there because of your clinical expertise, you will be expected to provide input in this area. In some interviews you may be directed by the chair to establish certain factors.

The main aim is to find out if the candidate has the necessary knowledge, skills and attributes for the post. Check through the information that the candidate has supplied on the application form or CV. It is usually unnecessary to question education or qualifications, unless there are ambiguities or irregularities in the application. Note down any other points you would like to clarify, or areas that you would like to expand upon. These notes will form the basis for your questions.

Think of direct questions that will elicit factual information; and open questions that will encourage more in-depth answers. Be especially careful to avoid leading questions. These tend to provide hints to the candidate on the expected answer. For example, 'We have strong links with the education department and several joint projects. What would you consider to be the main attributes of the post holder?' is likely to elicit a response on liaison skills.

Other questions can be directed at finding out:

- The reason they are applying for the post (this is particularly important if the move appears illogical, e.g. less money, lower grade)
- The reason they are leaving their present post

- ○ Their strengths
- ○ Their weaknesses now, and their potential weaknesses in regard to the post
- ○ Their personal qualities – reliability, personality, initiative, commitment
- ○ Any special qualities/experience/skills they would bring to the post
- ○ The candidate's future career plans.

Make sure you formulate your questions before the interview, and try them out on a colleague. Ask them if they were clear and unambiguous.

Questions with a practical bias or clinical scenarios need to be structured carefully. If there are too many ifs and buts, the candidate will have to ask a series of questions to clarify your question. Try answering the question yourself. If it takes more than a few minutes to answer, it should be re-phrased or dropped from your list.

Preparing your questions in this way will also prevent you from falling into the trap of the multiple question. This is when you ask several questions in one. These are very difficult for candidates to process and answer.

Remember the interview is also an opportunity to exchange information with the candidate. Be prepared to respond to her questions. You may also want to give some information about the organisation and department. Prepare a few main points and present these in a logical order.

Introductions

An easy start to the interview is for panel members to introduce themselves. A brief statement about themselves and why they are on the panel will suffice. This is preferable to the more formal style of the chair introducing members. The general aim is to relax the candidate.

Asking the questions

A few simple questions at the beginning of the interview will help the candidate to settle down and relax. It is only natural for them to be nervous at the beginning of the interview.

Avoid firing a series of unrelated questions at the candidate. These will make the interview disjointed and confrontational for the interviewee. Try to group questions that relate to a specific area together. Tell the candidate what sort of questions you are asking and why, and warn them when you are changing topic.

Evaluating the candidate

The most obvious way of evaluating the candidate is to study their responses to your questions. You need to listen not only to the content, but also to how the candidate answers. Do they avoid questions or seem to miss the point? Are their answers logical and well structured, or are they long and rambling? The face-to-face contact gives the opportunity to assess factors, like attitude and enthusiasm, which are hard to deduce from an application form.

In making this evaluation you need to be aware of any bias affecting your choice of candidate. It is a well-known phenomenon that interviewers tend to recruit people who are like themselves (Herriot 1989) – the mirror image syndrome. Other sources of bias are stereotypes particularly about age, sex, race, colour and disability (Pedler *et al.* 1994).

Recording

You need to have some written notes about each candidate. However, avoid taking these during the interview, as this is distracting and might inhibit the candidate. Arrange the appointments so that there is time in between to record relevant details, thoughts and opinions about the candidate.

Feedback

It is becoming standard practice for employers to give feedback to unsuccessful candidates. This helps the person develop their job search skills. It will also help you to formalise your decision making. The feedback should always be constructive, and highlight to the candidate their strengths as well as their particular shortcomings.

Summary Points

- One of the main roles of the manager is recruiting suitable staff for vacancies. This is achieved by advertising, shortlisting applications and inviting suitable candidates to interview.

- Traditional selection interviews focus on obtaining information from the candidate. There is little two-way interaction.

- An alternative approach is to encourage the candidate to take an active role in the selection process. There are advantages to this method for both parties.

- The first step in the selection process is to describe the nature of the post (job description), and identify the sort of qualities that are needed by the post holder (job specification). This information will be used by the human resources department to draw up a job advertisement.

- Send a job description and information package to applicants.

- Use the essential qualities listed on the job specification to shortlist candidates. You may want to refer to references before the interview, or make your own impressions first.

- Hold the interviews in a quiet room away from distractions and interruptions.

- Arrange for a member of staff to greet candidates and show them to the waiting area.

- The type of interview will affect the lay-out of the room and the interaction with the candidates.

- Prepare your questions before the interview. They need to be clear and unambiguous.

- The main aim is to find out if the candidate has the necessary knowledge, skills and attributes for the post.

- Use the interview to provide the candidate with some information. Prepare two or three main points.

- Study the candidate's responses to your questions. The way they answer is just as important as the content.

- Use the interview to assess factors such as attitude and enthusiasm.

- Be careful of any bias in your selection. One of the commonest is to recruit someone who is very similar to yourself.

- Provide feedback to unsuccessful candidates about their strengths and their shortcomings.

Applying for a post

Applying for a job is about selling yourself to the employer. You need to get yourself noticed, and then demonstrate that you fit the employer's requirements. You will be asked to complete an application form or send a curriculum vitae. The information in these documents will be used to determine your suitability for interview. Usually there will be four or five other candidates who will be shortlisted along with you. The interview is the final but crucial stage in your application. This section will show you the best way to present yourself at each stage in this process.

Writing a curriculum vitae

A curriculum vitae or CV is a record of your knowledge, skills, and employment history. It may be your first point of contact with your prospective employer, and therefore its presentation deserves close attention. Your CV is not a static document. It will reflect changes in your life. This does not mean that you simply add on each new episode of your career history. Most people from the middle of their career onwards will have had several jobs, received a wide range of in-service training, and accrued numerous skills. If you try to include all of this on one CV it will be overlong and lack impact.

It needs to be re-written each time you apply for a new post, the type and level of employment determining which information it is relevant to include. This is the advantage of the CV above the straightforward application form. First, it allows you to make a choice about the information you want to highlight to an employer. Second, you can decide the sequence in which you want to present information. This can have a crucial impact on whether you are selected.

One of the best pieces of advice I have been given about writing a CV is to make it look as if – 'you have been somewhere and you know where you are going'. Part of this is showing how you have built on your achievements. For example, you might want to emphasise how post graduate training enabled you to develop a specialism in your clinical field. The idea is that you have a plan, and that things have not just happened in a haphazard way. Be specific about your achievements. Statements like 'I am presently a radiologist at...' tell the interviewer nothing about you. This information is 'as read'. Instead write about your experience in supervision, budgeting, or specific clinical skills. Back this up with details of the number of staff, size of budget and type of caseload.

The job specification will indicate which activities are relevant. These are the ones to include on your CV. Always put the most important information at the beginning, and the least important at the end. This means starting with your strengths. A recent graduate with limited experience may want to stress her qualifications, including the specific grades and any special awards for outstanding achievements. Her education and qualification will come first. Somebody with excellent work experience but mediocre qualifications may want to place more weight on their employment history – educational background would only be mentioned briefly. A clinician applying for a management post may want to stress experience in staff supervision, or budgeting. Whatever you do always be truthful! This is about presenting your best side, not re-writing history.

Another way of making your CV more dynamic is to use active or doing words. Instead of writing, 'I was *responsible* for the hearing screening for the under fives'; write 'I *co-ordinated* the hearing screening for under fives'. Other active words to use in your CV are:

administer	develop	motivate
advise	design	organise
analyse	direct	plan
create	evaluate	problem-solve
communicate	implement	negotiate
construct	initiate	resolve
co-ordinate	liaise	supervise

Think of descriptive words that have impact. Here are some examples:

innovative	persistent	dynamic
creative	convincing	flexible

Remember to include any experience, skills or knowledge that are relevant to the post. These may not necessarily be something you have gained through work. If you have a current driving licence you can put this under personal details. The ability to speak other languages is always worth noting either under qualifications or special interests. Other examples of relevant skills are computer literacy, voluntary counselling work (e.g. Samaritans), public speaking skills.

Your CV also needs to say something about you as an individual. This will make you a more interesting candidate, and will provide the interviewer with some useful ideas for questions. Describe your interests, hobbies, activities, volunteer experience, or community activities. Include anything unusual that gives you an extra dimension and reveals something about you as a person. However, keep your responses brief. Compare these two examples:

Hobbies

Dancing. Sports. Reading.

Hobbies

Greek Dancing. Hang gliding. Member of a creative writing group.

Which one is more interesting? Which one makes you want to know more? There is no need to rush out and take up a dangerous sport. You can make your hobbies sound more interesting by giving specific information. A common hobby is cooking. This might involve inventing your own recipes, providing teas for the local cricket club, planning dinner parties or attending an evening course to learn a new style of cooking. Provide interesting detail rather than a bland umbrella term.

The style of your CV will vary according to the nature of the post, your background and experience. There are three main types:

- Recent trainee or graduate
- Chronological
- Functional.

All CVs start with some personal information about the applicant. At the very least you need to put your name, address, and a contact telephone number. Other optional details you may want to include are marital status, number of children, date of birth and nationality.

CHRONOLOGICAL CV

This is a standard format for a CV, which highlights accomplishments according to chronological order. Choose this style if you have a clear developmental pattern to your career.

Start with your education and qualifications. The amount of detail for this section is optional and depends on the stage you have reached in your career. If you have several postgraduate qualifications, the subjects and grades of your school certificates are less important.

Next, list each of your previous posts under the job title and employer with the relevant dates. The month and year will suffice. Start with your most recent post and work backwards. (If your last post was less than impressive, or you have had a period out of the job market you might want to consider the functional CV below.) For each of your jobs, briefly describe your responsibilities, specifying any outstanding achievements or developments. If you have stayed in one post for several years, you need to emphasise a progression in your experience and skills. This might be in developing a clinical specialism or an increase in responsibility. Highlight these developments by putting the date when your responsibilities changed and so on.

Other relevant headings include publications, research, and additional training. It may be more appropriate for you to list publications and research on a separate sheet, particularly if you have a long list.

The chronological CV illustrates clearly what you have done from school until the present. It is a particularly good style for highlighting continuity and developmental progression in your career. However, it does tend to show up any gaps in your employment or tendencies to job hop.

Here is an example of a chronological CV:

Maria Grech
Flat C
356 Wellington Avenue
Bridnorth
Stantonshire Tel No: 0223 091674

Date of Birth: 31/10/69
Age: 27 years

Education:
Bridnorth Comprehensive
(Sept. '80 – July '87)

7 GCSE
A levels (1987)
French (B) Biology (B) Sociology (C)

Post School Qualifications: BSc Speech Pathology (First Class)
(Stantonshire University Sept. '87 – July '91)

Current Post:
Mid Stantonshire Community Health Trust (since May '93) Specialist Speech and Language Therapist (Grade 2) Developing a specialist service for statemented children in mainstream. Initiating training programmes for education staff.

Previous post:
Easton Community Trust (Oct '91 – April '93) Generalist Speech and Language Therapist (Grade 1) Providing assessment and treatment for pre-school children attending nurseries and health centres.

Organising and running speech and language groups for school aged children.

Other Training:
Derbyshire Language Scheme; Makaton.

Hobbies and Interests:
Sailing. Learning Greek (Intermediate stage).

TRAINEE OR GRADUATE ENTRY

If you are a trainee or recent graduate you are unlikely to have any substantial work experience. The chronological CV is probably the best style for you, with an emphasis on your educational achievements and qualifications. If you have just completed a training course, you can include details of practical placements. Remember to highlight any experience that demonstrates you have skills or experience that are relevant to the post. Were you head of year? This would demonstrate you were a responsible person with leadership qualities. Were you a student representative? You will have experience of report writing, participating in committees, and working with a variety of people.

Here is an example of a graduate entry CV:

David Edwards
49 Tungate Drive
Easton
Garnley Tel No 0356 789 245
Age: 22

Education
King Edward High School, Nortonshire (1985–1992)

Qualifications:
GCSE (1990)
Maths (A) English Language (A) French (A) Chemistry (B) Biology (A)
Physics (C) Economics (B)

A levels (1992)
Biology (A) Chemistry (B) Physics (B)

Head boy 1990
Captain of the School Rugby team (1990–1992)

Post School Qualifications:
BSc Physiotherapy – 2:1
(Garnley University Sept.'92 – July '96)

Practical experience was gained on 10 placements of 100 hours each. Rotation included surgical, respiratory, neurological, care of the elderly and intensive care.

Hobbies and Interests:
Captain of the Garnley Amateur twelve-aside-football team. Local secretary for the real ale campaign.

FUNCTIONAL

A functional CV focuses on skills and experience. For example, a ward sister might record her skills, experience and achievements under the headings of nursing, budgeting, staff supervision, and administration. A summary of employment history is included after the list of functional experiences. This is a good style for people who want to emphasise work experience in several areas. It also highlights past as well as present strengths. However, it is not always as acceptable as the traditional chronological approach.

Here is an example of a functional CV:

Lisa O'Brien (Mrs)
The Honeypot Cottage
Furze Lane
Poreton Village
Landsbury Tel No: 223 45789

Areas of Major Experience

Health Visitor: Using a holistic approach to working with
                             the elderly. Promoting independent living.
                             Providing support, information and advice
                             to carers.

Training: Development of programmes to raise awareness about the health problems of smoking and drinking for the elderly. Training student nurses in the diseases of the elderly population.

Committee work: Establishing local branch of Cruise. Member of the steering committee for Crossroads. Initiatives in raising funds from social services.

Employment History:

1977–1978   Staff Nurse
(Landsbury General Infirmary)
Surgical ward.

1978–1979   Staff Nurse
(Royal Horington Hospital)
Geriatric ward.

1980–1985   General Health Visitor
(Horington Health Authority)
Advice and support to families with under fives. Participation in a multi-disciplinary audiology clinic for screening hearing.

Current Post:

Health Visitor to the Elderly (Horington Community Trust) (since 1990)
Providing a specialist service to the elderly, which involves close liaison with local voluntary organisations.

Education:
O level: English, Maths, Biology, Home Economics

Post School Qualifications
1976 State Registered Nurse
1977 Joint Board course (Elderly)
1980 Diploma of Health Visiting

Professional Memberships Registered Member of the United Kingdom Central Council for Nursing, Midwifery and health visiting

Interests Creating novelty cake decorations. Member of the Horington women's hockey team.

Type your CV on good quality A4 paper. Never send a photocopy (Goodworth 1979). It needs to be succinct with a maximum length of two pages.

Experiment with different lay-outs, until you are satisfied the information is clearly presented. Emphasise headings in bold text, and use spaces rather than boxes to separate different sections. (Boxes break up the text, and make it harder to read.)

Always have a final check of accuracy, grammar and spelling. Keep a copy of your CV with the original job advertisement.

References

Approach your referees well ahead of the date of the interview. Provide them with a copy of your completed application form or CV, and a copy of the job description and job specification. This will help them in making the reference relevant to the post. Names and addresses of referees are usually provided on a separate piece of paper.

Application forms

Many employers require candidates to complete an application form. These consist of a standard set of questions, that each candidate is required to complete in the same way.

There is usually a section where candidates are invited to provide any further information in support of their application. This is the most important part of the form. Never write a one liner. Use this section to highlight your achievements and experience, and say why you want the post. This section can be prepared in a similar way to your CV. Select specific examples of your skills or experience that match the requirements outlined in the job specification. Write these in the form of a personal statement. Choose active words from the list above to make your statement more dynamic. Make sure that all the information you give is accurate and up to date.

Type or hand write your application form with an ink pen not biro, and keep a copy of your completed form with the original advertisement.

Dressing for the interview

People *do* make judgements about people on the basis of their clothing and physical appearance. Usually this happens within the first thirty seconds of meeting them. Whether we agree with this or not, it is necessary to put some thought into preparing yourself for the interview. Even if your post involves your wearing a uniform or casual clothing, interviewers will be expecting you to 'make an effort'. At the very least you are showing the interviewers that you are taking the interview seriously. Here are some tips for men and women:

General appearance

The main requirement of any candidate is to appear well-groomed and clean. This means freshly pressed clothes and clean shoes.

Hair

Invest in a hair cut a few days before the interview. Note I have used the word cut as opposed to re-style. You do not want to find yourself with a disastrous hair style that will make you feel awful. Long hair needs to be tied back.

Clothes

Whatever you wear, it needs to be comfortable. Loose clothing is generally better than tightly fitted garments. Choose materials suitable for the weather. There is no need to buy an outfit especially for your interview, unless your wardrobe is completely bare. In fact it is better if you have worn the clothes before. This way you will know how much the material creases, whether your skirt rides up or how hot you feel in your suit after a few hours. Women need to take a spare pair of tights.

Shoes

These need to be clean and repaired before the interview. No worn down heels. Women are usually recommended to wear shoes with a small heel rather than flat shoes or stilettos. Men need to avoid large cowboy boots or other types of footwear that are too large for their trousers to fit over comfortably.

Accessories

For women, the wearing of a few discreet pieces of jewellery, and a good quality scarf or belt can transform an outfit. Less is usually best, with extremes of size, length and colour avoided. The 'mobility factor' of your accessories is a good test of their suitability. If your ear-rings dangle and your scarf flows out behind you like a flag, then leave them at home.

Men need to think about their ties, belts and socks. Ties should reach to the waistband, no lower and no higher. Colours and patterns need to be restrained. Invest in a good quality leather belt with a small, neat buckle.

Choose socks in the same colour as your shoes or trousers. Definitely no red or white ones.

Smell

This refers to perfume, aftershave and strong smelling soaps. Smell is a very individual sense. What you think is wonderful, may be a rotten egg for somebody else. Choose toiletry items that have a light scent.

Image

Suits project authority. They are the ideal choice for both men and women. If you have a limited budget then a good quality jacket that fits well is the next choice. Team it with items of clothing in co-ordinating tones. It will be impossible to get an exact match on the colour, and any slight differences will only emphasise you are wearing odd garments. In the summer women can opt for a dress as an acceptable alternative to the suit, but again this needs a jacket. Unfortunately it is still not advisable for women to wear trousers to an interview.

Fashion extremes are fine if you are applying for a job in a design studio, but tend to be less acceptable for posts in the health service. *You* need to be noticed, not your clothes. Choose dark neutral colours that suit you. (Appropriate colours would include black, charcoal, dark brown, navy, olive green, bronze.) Avoid wearing black if it gives your skin the pallor of a ghost. Wear a different colour, or use a bright colour around the neckline.

Women in revealing necklines or short skirts tend to project less authority. If you want to wear a shorter style, then choose skirts that rest just above the knee when you sit down. Wear a necklace with an open neckline. Consider wearing a slip if your skirt is unlined.

Men need to be aware of their trouser lengths. Large expanses of hairy shin are off-putting. Check the gap between socks and trousers when you sit down.

*   *   *   *   *   *

The main thing to remember is to be yourself and to feel comfortable. Choose an outfit that you know suits you. Definitely avoid anything you have worn to unsuccessful interviews.

The interview

Being punctual is essential. Do a dummy run of your journey, ideally at a similar time of day to your interview. If you are travelling away from home, ask friends who know the city for some advice. The relevant personnel department will also be able to help, and may have information about where to stay overnight. A street map will be invaluable. Check the times of trains and buses, even if you have used them before. Time-tables are changed on a regular basis and alterations due to engineering works are frequent.

Arrive ten minutes early so you can freshen up and relax before the interview. You want your appearance to be neat and professional; so leave extraneous coats and bags with a secretary.

First impressions are lasting (Arvey and Campion 1984). What does your non-verbal communication say about you? How will you enter the room? Shoulders bowed and head down. Or with your head up and shoulders back. The second posture will exude confidence. This will be reinforced by looking and smiling at the interviewer. Handshakes are important. People have strong reactions to touch, and although it is a common form of greeting, it is also an intimate gesture. A limp fish is off-putting, and a bone crusher is annoying. A brief but firm handshake is best.

Use your body language to emit positive signals. Maintain an erect posture once you are sitting. Show that you are interested by sitting forwards slightly, and leaning towards the interviewers. Look interested and show you are listening by nodding your head.

Respond to questions positively. This is your opportunity to sell yourself. The way that you answer questions will influence the selectors as much as what you say. Take a few seconds to think of your response. You want to give as full an answer as possible, and to present it coherently. The silence will not be as long as you think. Keep your replies brief and to the point. Never avoid answering a question. This will look very suspicious.

Use your responses to show that you know how to do the job, and that you have the necessary experience. The interviewer will often provide you with prompts, like 'Tell me about your experiences at the health centre, and describe how you feel they are relevant to this vacancy'. Sometimes you will need to think of ways that you can introduce information, but do not do this at the expense of answering the question.

Always give specific examples of what you have done. Avoid statements like 'I did similar work at Honely Health Centre'. Instead describe exactly what you did, for example 'I set up a very successful drop-in clinic at Honely Health Centre', or 'I provided educational talks for local schools on dental hygiene.' Your answers need to have a blend of facts and feelings (Roberts 1985). Say if you really enjoyed something.

The interviewer may describe a scenario and ask how you would respond in this situation. This could be on any aspect of the job, but is usually a query about clinical areas. Always respond using the first person, and if possible give examples of similar problems you have dealt with before. If possible try to compare your different experiences to show that you have thought about them.

Like your CV your responses must demonstrate that you have the skills relevant to the post. If flexibility is an important quality, you can provide examples of how you have coped with change.

Be prepared to respond to questions about why you want the job. Show the interviewer that you know something about their organisation. They will be flattered if you demonstrate that you have selected them as a potential employer. Build on your replies to questions – 'I enjoy the training aspect of my present post. I am attracted to this vacancy, because of the involvement in in-service training'. Remember the interview is an opportunity for you to decide whether you want the post. This may be your only chance if there was no informal interview. Aim to find out about:

- the details of the post
- the department
- the organisation
- the type and amount of supervision or support
- training opportunities
- career development.

It may be necessary to do some probing. Find out exactly what is required of the post holder. A statement like 'you are expected to work such hours as are reasonably necessary to fulfil your duties' needs to be investigated. What exactly does this mean? What sort of hours will you be expected to work?

End the interview on a positive note. This is the time to say if you are very interested in the post (Heylin 1991). A polite 'Thank you for seeing me' or 'It has been very interesting hearing about your department' will leave the interviewers with a good impression.

Feedback

If you fail to be selected for the post, you need to get feedback as to why. This will help you to prepare for your next interview. It is also human nature to want to know the reason. You need to get specific feedback from the selection panel.

Checklist for preparing for interviews

Research

☐ You have made an informal visit.

Or

☐ You have discussed the post with the relevant manager.

☐ You have read the relevant material relating to the organisation and its aims, philosophies and objectives.

☐ You have read the job description thoroughly.

Applications

☐ You have contacted your referees.

☐ Your CV is updated.

☐ You have completed all the sections on the application form.

☐ You have signed and dated it.

☐ You have written a covering letter.

☐ You have made a copy of your CV/application form.

Preparation

☐ You have prepared responses to possible interview questions.

☐ You have prepared questions to ask the interviewers.

☐ You have identified examples of your work that relate to the requirements of the post.

Interview

☐ You have checked your travel arrangements.

☐ You have selected an appropriate outfit which is clean and pressed ready for the interview.

☐ You have collected any relevant documents to take to the interview.

Action points

Use the following points to help you to prepare your application.

(1) Find out all the information you can about the post for which you are applying. Use the information that the employer has sent to you (job description, job specification, advertisement, job package). Supplement this with any advice you can glean from colleagues who have a similar post. What sort of person do *you* think will suit this post?

(2) List the knowledge, skills and experience required by the employer. How do you compare with these? What are your strengths and weaknesses in relation to these areas?

(3) What evidence or examples do you have of your knowledge, skills and experience? This might be educational attainment, a professional qualification, or past responsibilities. You need to show the employer what you have done that reflects the level of experience required by the post.

(4) Make a list of your achievements. Make these as specific as possible. Note down what you did and when you did it. What was the result of your achievement?

Here are some tips on preparing for the actual interview.

(5) Try to anticipate the interviewer's questions and prepare responses. Here are some common interview questions:

- What do you feel you have to offer this department; authority; hospital?
- What are your strengths?
- What are your weaknesses?
- Why are you interested in this position?
- What are your long term career plans?
- This post involves…(working as a team; travelling; night shifts; dealing with violent patients; etc.). How will you cope with this?
- What were your main achievements in your last post?

- What personal qualities do you think you have that will contribute to this post?
- Why do you want to leave your present post?
- What were the major problems in your last job? Tell me how you dealt with one of these problems.
- How do you see your previous work experience contributing to this post?

Test your replies out on a friend. What is his reaction?

(6) Enlist the help of friends in role playing the interview. Have one as the interviewer and another as an observer. Judging your own performance can be very hard to do. Ask your friends to give you feedback. If possible video record yourself. Use this checklist to rate yourself.

☐ You entered the room with a confident manner.

☐ You gave eye-contact to the interviewer.

☐ You remembered to smile.

☐ Your handshake was firm but brief.

☐ You sat up straight, leaning forwards slightly.

☐ You nodded and looked interested when the interviewer was talking.

☐ Your response to questions was positive.

☐ You answered all the questions.

☐ You answered questions in full.

☐ Your responses were succinct.

☐ You gave specific examples of your achievements.

☐ You demonstrated that you knew something about the employer.

☐ You stated why you wanted the post.

☐ You asked appropriate questions.

☐ You ended the interview with a positive comment.

Summary points – applying for a post

- There are two main ways that you can sell yourself to the interviewer – your curriculum vitae (CV) or the application form, and the interview.

- A curriculum vitae or CV is a record of your knowledge, skills, and employment history.

- Make your CV relevant to the post for which you are applying. Write it using active or doing words, and provide specific examples of your achievements.

- The style of your CV will vary according to the nature of the post, your background and experience. There are three main types – recent trainee or graduate, chronological or functional.

- If you are required to complete an application form, make sure it is accurate and that you have answered all the questions.

- Always provide a full response in the section inviting you to add further information to support your application.

- The interviewer will expect you to make an effort with your dress. Clothes need to be neat, clean and tidy.

- Punctuality is essential. Check out your travel details.

- First impressions are lasting. Enter the room with a confidant posture, looking at the interviewer and smiling. Use a firm handshake.

- Use your body language to show you are interested and enthusiastic.

- Respond to questions in a positive manner. Answer all the questions as fully as possible. Keep your replies brief.

- Give specific examples of your achievements.

- Show the interviewer that you know something about the job.

- Prepare some questions to ask about the post and the organisation.

- End the interview on a positive note.

- Ask for feedback if you are unsuccessful.

Interviewing Skills in Context
Grievance and Disciplinary Interviews

A *grievance* is a complaint brought by an employee against a colleague or senior member of staff. This might relate to the conduct, performance or attitude of this person.

A *disciplinary* matter arises when an employee behaves in an inappropriate way. This might relate to their conduct, performance or attitude.

It is standard practice to have published procedures for both grievance and disciplinary matters. These are usually made available to all employees through an induction package. These procedures should be read thoroughly if you are involved in either bringing a grievance, or in disciplining a member of your staff. You will see from the information that the interview is only part of these procedures. However, it is still a core element.

Factors affecting communication in the interview

Due to the content of the interview there is always a strong emotional element. These are likely to cover a range of feelings that include:

- embarrassment
- anger
- fear
- frustration
- disbelief
- shock.

Feelings may be combined into a potent mixture. Anger and fear are common reactions which, mixed together, often produce explosive results. Participants need to be aware of this factor, as their style of interaction can either defuse or exacerbate the situation.

It is not always possible to predict what people will be feeling. You might expect an employee to feel embarrassed about being disciplined, rather than the manager who has brought the disciplinary charge. However, it may be the manager who feels embarrassed about having to take such an action, and the employee who feels angry.

Have you ever been disciplined? Have you ever brought a grievance against your manager? Even if you have never been involved in a formal case, there are probably times when you felt you were dealt with unjustly. How did you feel? How did it affect your working relationship with these people?

The other factor to be aware of in these situations is the need for both parties to maintain a communication channel. Often a grievance or disciplinary matter is a result of a breakdown in communication. This is why most procedures have a process of arbitration, where the parties must show that they have met and attempted to resolve the issues. Problems should never be stored up until a member of staff is summoned to a disciplinary hearing, or feelings of resentment suppressed until a formal complaint is made.

Arranging the venue

The interview needs to be held away from the participants' normal place of work. This avoids the possibility of any embarrassing encounters between participants and colleagues. It is also difficult to maintain privacy if an adjoining room is being used by a colleague. A room in the human resources department is a good choice.

Due to the nature of the interview it is best that the room is arranged with some formality. It needs to signal the gravity of the situation. This is not to say that the interviewee should be made to feel as if they were in an interrogation. It is useful if there is somewhere for people to place their papers, either by seating people around a table or providing each party with a small side table.

Preparation

Both parties need to prepare thoroughly before the interview. This is only possible if the purpose of the interview has been made clear. Occasionally one side will try to outfox the other by obscuring the exact content of the meeting. This is in the hope of gaining a winning edge from their opponent's lack of preparation. This is bad practice, and is likely to increase any feelings of anger or injustice.

If you are called to a meeting, try to establish the agenda, even if you are not told the details. As an employee you are obliged to attend a meeting called by your manager – otherwise, you are in breach of your contract.

The preparation is very similar for a grievance and a disciplinary meeting. It consists of gathering relevant facts and planning a logical presentation. You need to prepare an exact description of the incident or incidents. This description will detail when and where it happened, and any information about the relevant circumstances. It makes your case stronger if you have witnesses to the incident. However, people are often reluctant to come forward, especially if asked to support a grievance.

Organising the interview

In this type of interview a chairperson is invaluable, and may even be a stipulation of your procedures. Ideally this person will be someone who is perceived by both parties as neutral, and is not involved in the decision making. You may use a representative, but they may be seen as less than impartial by employees. Alternatively, a member of a different department could be enlisted. This is perfectly acceptable so long as they are not someone who works alongside any of the key participants.

The role of the chair is to deal with procedural issues. They control the flow of communication by indicating who speaks when. Insist on participants 'going through the chair', which means that participants must request permission from the chair to make a statement. This takes the heat out of the interaction by slowing down the pace. Comments are then made directly to the chair rather than to the other members. This is a highly stylised form of interaction, but is a very effective way of avoiding heated arguments.

The other consideration is the timing of the interview. Is the interviewee likely to be able to concentrate, if they have to return to work after the interview? Try to organise these types of interviews for later in the afternoon.

Grievance interviews

Interviewee

In a grievance interview the main facts need to be presented in detail. If you have done your homework, you will already have a plan for your presentation.

Present your evidence clearly and logically. Start by stating your grievance in one or two succinct phrases. Then recount the sequence of events using specific examples to support your arguments. If possible, relate your comments to organisational policies, for example policies regarding discrimination.

Structure your evidence so that related items are grouped together. This prevents the discussion deteriorating into a string of accusations 'And he said that...' and 'Oh yeah that's another thing'.

The nature of a grievance is such that feelings often run very high. Try to keep your emotions under control, as you are more likely to be taken seriously. Remain calm and present your comments in a firm tone. Your aim is to show your employer that you have absolutely no doubts that you have a fair case.

Interviewer

Your main aim is to establish the facts of the grievance. Show the employee that you take it seriously and want to find out all the details.

Allow the interviewee time to express their feelings and concerns. It is important that you listen carefully to their comments. If necessary, clarify any unclear points, but avoid asking too many questions at this stage (Croner 1985).

Once the interviewee has finished presenting their case, more directive questions can be used to establish specific details. Ask for examples if these have not been provided. Make sure that you have a full understanding of the interviewee's case. Summarise the grievance to check you have all the facts.

How the interview is concluded depends on your evaluation of the situation. Whatever the outcome it is important to express the decision in a neutral fashion. See the advice below in the disciplinary section on communication styles.

Disciplinary interview

Interviewee

It is very important that you are given specific examples of the behaviour that has precipitated the disciplinary hearing. If you have not been fully briefed before the meeting you must elicit the information from the interviewer. Use closed questions to get specific details. You need information on four things:

- A description of the conduct, performance or attitude that has been found to be inappropriate
- The dates and times when this happened
- The person or persons who witnessed these behaviours
- The standards, rules or regulations these behaviours have breached.

You can decide on your response once you know what the case is against you. How you deal with it will depend on whether you think the criticisms are valid or not. Do you agree that these behaviours occurred? Were the standards or regulations that you broke communicated to you clearly? The other thing to consider is whether there were any extenuating circumstances. It is important to make it clear to your employers if anything has prevented you from performing your work. This might be illness, personal problems or even living conditions.

Your main challenge is to control your emotions. You may be feeling afraid, angry, confused or a mixture of these emotions. You need to stay calm. If you are agitated, you will be less able to listen and plan your responses. Remember you are entitled to have a representative from your union or a friend who can help you present your case.

Interviewer

You need to make sure that the employee understands the nature of the disciplinary matter. This means making sure they know what they have done and when they did it. Describe the incident exactly. You also need to make clear what standards of behaviour were expected, and how these were communicated to the employee. It is important to show that the employee should have known the appropriate behaviour expected by his employers. Avoid any ambiguities in interpretation, as this might be crucial if the employee appeals against the decision.

If you have questions for the employee, ask them one at a time. Too many together will sound like an interrogation. Try to establish if there were any extenuating circumstances.

Some people view the disciplinary process as a way of meting out punishment – the disciplinary is an end in itself. The alternative is to use the situation to problem solve with the employee. An action plan can then be agreed upon and set into motion.

Your communication style will play a significant role in the interview. One way of examining your interaction is the transactional analysis approach suggested by Berne (1964). This proposes that individuals have three characteristic ways of behaving. Berne calls these ego states.

They are:

> The *parent* who responds with behaviours similar to those used by parents or other authority figures during childhood. These may be supportive, punitive, or controlling.

The *child* who exhibits curiosity and enthusiasm. They may also, like all children, alternate between naughtiness and an anxiety to please.

The *adult* whose behaviour is based on logic and reasoned argument.

Breakdowns in communication often occur when there is a mismatch between the ego states of the participants. If one person responds as a parent, the other is likely to respond as the child. The manager may feel they have succeeded if they elicit the child who wants to please. However, the response to the parent is more likely to be the naughty child. Look at these different examples. Do you recognise the different ego states?

(1) 'I'm your manager. I tell you what to do. You do it.'

'Well, it's a pity you don't know what the hell you're talking about then.'

(2) 'How can we sort this problem out?'

'I am happy to do whatever you suggest. Whatever you say, I'll be onto it right away.'

(3) 'You're complaining you haven't received your travel expenses. What about all the times you've been late this month?'

'I am happy to discuss my time-keeping with you at a separate meeting. I am concerned that my travel expenses are outstanding by three months.'

In a disciplinary interview responding as an adult is likely to reduce any potential conflict.

Summary Points

- A *grievance* is a complaint brought by an employee against a colleague or senior member of staff. This might relate to the conduct, performance or attitude of this person.

- A *disciplinary* matter arises when an employee behaves in an inappropriate way. This might relate to their conduct, performance or attitude.

- It is standard practice to have a published set of procedures relating to grievance or disciplinary matters. Read these carefully before your interview.

- There is a high emotional content to these types of interviews. Your style of communication will affect how much these feelings interfere with the interaction.

- Remember to keep communication channels open with the participants. Never store things up until the interview.

- Arrange to use a room away from the participants usual place of work. This provides a neutral atmosphere and avoids any potential embarrassment caused by meeting colleagues.

- Prepare thoroughly. Make sure that you have a complete agenda before the meeting, so that you can gather relevant facts and plan your presentation.

- A neutral chairperson is invaluable for structuring the interaction.

- In a grievance interview the emphasis is on the interviewee expressing their complaint. The interviewer will spend a greater amount of time listening.

- In a disciplinary interview the emphasis is on making clear what the breach of conditions has been. This includes reiterating for the interviewee the standards to which they have failed to adhere.

Interviewing Skills in Context
Interviews with the Media

Occasionally health professionals are requested by the press, radio or television to provide information or give opinions on current health care topics. Normally this is an experience that very few health professionals encounter in their working life. It is natural therefore for you to experience a mixture of feelings, that will include anxiety, if you are approached to appear on the radio or television.

Before accepting any invitation there are a number of safeguards you need to take. Always make sure that you get clearance from your manager and talk to your public relations department. Are you complying with your employer's guidelines on contacts with the media? It is your responsibility to ensure that you have the expertise to answer the questions and provide the necessary information. It may be more appropriate to pass the interviewer to another colleague.

Find out which organisation the interviewer is representing, and ask for an office telephone number where you can ring and check their identity. Establish when the interview will start. You may be surprised to find that comments made over the phone are used by a reporter. A radio interviewer may even be recording you.

Once you are satisfied that you are dealing with a genuine reporter, you need to find out what information they require and how it will be used. Does the programme have any particular angle or bias? The questions you are asked will give you a clue as to the likely slant that the interview will take.

If your job is likely to require you to meet regularly with the media, then training is essential.

Preparing for the interview

It is essential to prepare thoroughly for the interview. Before deciding what you will say, you need to find out as much as possible about the actual interview. You should expect to be told which programme you will appear in, and the aim of the interview. Do your own research by watching or listening to the programme.

What is the programme trying to achieve? Is it a help line, community action slot, or a scientific series? This will give you some idea of the type of questions you may be asked, and what information the presenters are seeking. Do they want medical facts, practical suggestions for health care or opinions on government policy? Knowing something about the usual style of the programme will help you to choose appropriate material and prepare responses. Find out about the target audience. This will help you find items that are of both interest and use to the viewers and listeners.

Ask for questions in advance and prepare responses to these and any others you think may occur. It is particularly important to try to anticipate questions for phone-ins, which demand quick answers with little time for thinking. It may not be possible for the interviewer to give you all the questions, so try to agree on one or two to open the interview.

As with any other interview, you need to find out when it will start and where it will take place. Check your travel arrangements and try to arrive early so details can be finalised. You will also need some time to relax.

What is your key message?

The bulk of your preparation will be in the content of your interview. Decide what your key message will be. Do not prepare a 'speech' or try to use a script. Keep to a few main points. Once you have chosen your message you can think about how you can say this within the available time slot.

Keep the information simple and avoid jargon, but be careful not to patronise either the interviewer or the audience. Remember 'never underestimate either the basic ignorance of your interviewers or their general intelligence and skill' (Breakwell 1990). Practise expressing your key message using a variety of words and phrases. Choose the best one. Repeat this process for your other main points.

You may be asked to give your opinion on a subject even though you were not given prior warning. So give some thought to potential questions in your preparation.

During the interview

Make sure the interviewer is clear about your name, title, your employer and where you work. Try to be as natural as possible whilst remaining clear and precise. Long and convoluting sentences are difficult for an audience to follow, so aim to be concise. Brief interviews demand even more precision in discussing the points, as there is no time for complex arguments.

Some interviewers have a hidden agenda and may try to side-track you onto other issues. Remain calm. Keep to your objectives, and be consistent. Learn to say what you want to say whatever the questions (Heylin 1991).

In a pre-recorded interview you may be asked questions that seem very similar. This is because the final edited version will have mixed and matched the questions and answers. Ask if you can see the final version and correct any misrepresentations.

Always protect confidentiality and get the written permission of any clients you may refer to in your interview. It may be necessary to change details such as gender, age and occupation to disguise the identity.

Be ready to give contact names and addresses of any relevant organisations. Have some practical suggestions or quick tips you can use if asked.

What is your body language saying?

On television the language of your body is just as important as your verbal language. We all know of cases where the interviewee has given shifty sideways glances or takes quick comic peeps at the camera. Generally it is best to concentrate on the interviewer.

Tone of voice, facial expression and posture need to match the content of your message. Concentrating on what you are going to say next can make you forget about smiling or sounding enthusiastic. Keep your posture as relaxed and open as possible. Crossed arms and half turning away suggest you are on the defensive. Fiddling and grooming gestures, like smoothing hair down, will make you appear nervous.

Group interviews

As with an individual interview it is important to find out the purpose of the interview and who else will be participating. Some group interviews have a rigid structure, with members contributing only when directed by the interviewer. Others adopt a more informal style of debate with the interviewer occasionally prompting changes in topic, or drawing participants into the discussion.

During the interview it is important to listen and look at the other interviewees. You may need to respond to their comments or modify your contribution. In a heated debate it can sometimes be difficult to get your chance to speak. Breakwell (1990) suggests using the following strategies. Try to get the presenter's attention by getting eye-contact or calling his or her name. If this fails to work, you can interrupt another interviewee when they pause. Start making your point in a firm and calm manner. Avoid using passive words like 'maybe' or 'perhaps', as they are unlikely to make an impact.

Image

One thing that may concern you about a televised interview is your appearance. This is not a trivial matter of vanity. The audience will make assumptions about your personality, background, education, and even your professional competence from your clothes and general appearance. Is your image communicating a different message from the one you intended? The wrong clothes and accessories can be distracting and interfere with the audience's ability to attend to what you are saying.

You can check this for yourself by watching interviews on the television. An interesting game is to try and guess the job or political persuasion of an interviewee when they are introduced. Are your predictions borne out during the interview?

The nature of the medium also dictates certain dress rules. Large metal jewellery may reflect the studio lights and certain colours and patterns can cause visual problems, for example red can look blurred around the edges.

Remember the following do's and don'ts:

Do:

- Wear loose, comfortable clothing
- Choose light materials or have removable layers (studio lights can get very hot)
- Go for simple patterns and designs
- Choose outfits in a single colour or shades of the same colour
- Get hair trimmed.

Don't:

- Wear bright reds
- Wear checks, herringbones or stripes
- Have large pieces of jewellery, (especially ear-rings) or noisy bracelets
- Choose extremes of colour or have strong contrasts, e.g. black and white.

Action Points

(1) Watch and listen to other health professionals being interviewed. Note the responses you found interesting and informative. How did they deal with criticism? How did they avoid using jargon? What responses were less successful? Did they let themselves be side-tracked? What questions led up to this?

(2) Prepare responses to common questions you are asked about your job. These might be in relation to specific illnesses or to health care in general.

(3) Prepare responses to the most awkward questions you may be asked. Think about how you might respond to provocative comments.

(4) Practise your interview with a colleague. Ask them to rate the content on interest, information, and clarity. Compare this with one practised on a friend with no health care experience.

Summary Points

- Check that the reporter is bona fide.

- Get clearance from your manager and the public relations department.

- Find out all you can about the interviewer and the programme. Is there any particular angle the media are taking?

- Guard against 'off the cuff' comments being used by the interviewer.

- Ask for questions in advance and prepare responses.

- Choose your key message. Identify two or three main points.

- Be natural. Do not use a prepared script.

- Keep your message simple and to the point. Avoid jargon. Make it informative and interesting.

- Protect the confidentiality of your clients.

- Do not allow yourself to be side-tracked. Be consistent in what you are saying.

- Remember to use body language that matches your message.

- Image is important in television interviews.

PART THREE

Professional Meetings

12 Preparation

13 Communication Roles

14 Presenting Self

15 Meetings Skills in Context:

    15.1   Business Meetings

    15.2   Multi-disciplinary Teams

    15.3   Case Conferences

    15.4   Committees

    15.5   Working Parties

Professional Meetings

Meetings, love them or loathe them, are an integral part of working life. They range from the ten minute chat with a colleague to the large annual general meeting. These meetings provide a structured forum for people to gather and share information. They are also a way for people to work together towards a common purpose.

The health professional will be involved in many different types of meetings. Some of these will focus on the care and management of the client, while others are administrative in function. Here are some examples:

- Representative on the *committee* of a local voluntary organisation
- Attending a *staff* meeting
- Chairing an *inter-departmental meeting*
- Participating in a *multidisciplinary team meeting*
- Attending a *case conference*.

Organising and chairing meetings requires a considerable amount of preparation and skill. Even participating as an ordinary member demands a certain level of competence in debating and discussion.

The main part of this section looks at the general skills required for meetings. It includes the following topics:

Preparation
Preparing for a meeting. Finding the right venue. Checklist for preparation.

Communication roles
How to prepare an agenda. The skill of chairing a meeting. Writing the minutes. Effective participation.

Presenting Self
Why you need to take meetings seriously. How to present yourself effectively.

The final part of this section looks at different kinds of meetings. Use these chapters for specific advice regarding meetings in these contexts:

Business Meetings

Why do we need a business meeting? Small groups versus large groups. Evaluating your meeting.

Multi-disciplinary Teams

How to organise a team meeting. Building a working relationship. Avoiding conflict. Checklist for a successful team.

Case Conferences

Presenting information in a case conference.

Committees

What are committees all about? Participating as a member. Chairing a committee.

Working Parties

Stages in problem solving. Contributing to a working party.

12

Preparation

All meetings require a certain amount of preparation. The complexity of this preparation depends on the formality and size of the meeting. This section concentrates on how to arrange and organise a meeting.

Time-tabling meetings

The first thing that the you need to think about is when to hold the meeting. Sometimes this is decided for you – for instance, if the department has always held a meeting on a Wednesday morning. At other times you will need to choose the best time.

The obvious criterion is the availability of the members. To ensure this you need to give notice of the meeting well in advance of the date. A large meeting may need to be announced several months ahead, whereas a date for a smaller internal meeting may only need a week's notice.

There are certain times of the year to avoid. These are around the major holiday periods, particularly during July and August. Half-term can also create problems if you have staff who work during term time only.

The time of day is also important. Avoid periods when people are less energetic, such as immediately after lunch. Motivation is not likely to be high last thing on a Friday or first thing on a Monday morning.

Sometimes you will be bound by the needs of your guest speakers. You will have to time-table your meeting to suit their requirements. Try to give them a slot at the beginning or end of your meeting, as this is less disruptive.

Deciding on membership

It is vital that the right people are at the meeting. It is surprising how often this point is forgotten. Decide who you think is necessary for the meeting. Your choice of participants will depend on the purpose of the meeting. Some people will be invited because of their position; others because of their particular expertise.

Circulating the agenda

You need to communicate the time, date and place of the meeting. These details are usually included on the agenda, which must be circulated to all members before the meeting. The agenda is a statement about the purpose and the content of the meeting. It consists of a list of items for discussion (see 'Communication roles' for a discussion on how to set the agenda). Members will find it useful if you include both the start and finish times, and any breaks for refreshments.

If appropriate, send travel details with the agenda. These should include a photocopy of a simple but adequate map, which has the venue clearly marked. Provide information about road, bus and rail links. However, it is not advisable to give specific times as these are subject to regular alteration. Instead provide the bus numbers and the names of local rail stations. It is essential you check information before it is sent out.

In some instances members will be required to study papers in preparation for the meeting. Send these with the agenda. Be careful not to send reams of paperwork. This will only put people off, and is a costly and time-consuming exercise. Instead, consider giving a précis of information.

Some organisers send the minutes of the previous meeting along with the agenda. This completely defeats the object of the minute taking system. Minutes help to define the actions that need to be implemented between meetings. It is essential therefore that they are circulated immediately after the previous meeting, and not just before the next one.

Venue

One of the key aspects of organising a meeting is arranging for a suitable venue. You may have facilities on site or you may wish to book accommodation elsewhere. 'Away days' are becoming increasingly popular. You will find your requirements grow in relation to the size and formality of the meeting. There are a number of factors to consider before making your choice.

Location

Choose a venue that is easy for all the members to reach. Ideally it will be situated close to public transport routes and have good access by road. Car parking facilities are a definite bonus.

Facilities

Find out what facilities are being offered. Are there phones, fax and photocopier machines? Check out what audio-visual equipment is available, and if there is on site technical support.

Size

It is important that the room is the right size for the number of participants. It will be uncomfortable if too many people are crammed into a small room. On the other hand a small number of people will feel lost in an oversized room.

Shape

The best shape for a meeting's room is rectangular. This ensures that everyone is able to see and be seen.

Seating

It is vital to get this right. People will soon lose interest in the meeting, if their bottom has gone to sleep! Chairs need to provide support for the back, but also need to have some cushioning particularly in the seat area. Of course, there need to be enough for all the participants with a few extra for any unexpected guests.

Room set-up

This will depend on the purpose of your meeting and the size of the group. Do you need tables for members to work on paper work? A large board room table allows each member some writing space.

At a large meeting you will need several rows of chairs. Avoid long straight rows; a curved arrangement is much better. Make sure there is plenty of aisle space.

People need to have a certain amount of personal space. Each person must have at least elbow room between themselves and the next person. There must also be space for people to move around. Is there space around the outside of the seating area? How easy is it for people to get to their seats?

Lighting

Choose a room with adequate lighting and preferable some natural light from a window. Check whether the lighting is controllable? Can it be dimmed? Are there spot lights?

Temperature

Avoid extremes of heat and cold. What facilities are there for heating or air-conditioning in the room? It is better if you have some control over these systems. A sudden improvement in the weather can raise both the room and the members to boiling point if the heating is on pre-set levels. Similar problems occur with over rigorous air-conditioning that leaves everybody shivering. Some form of ventilation is important, even if this is just being able to open a window.

Rooms with windows that are south facing can be a problem in the summer. Blinds are essential to keep out the glare of the sun, but do little to keep the room cool. You may be able to get round the problem if you book your meeting early in the morning when the sun is less hot. Generally it is better to avoid these rooms altogether.

Decor

Choose a room with a neutral scheme that uses pale creams and muted pastels. Carpets, curtains and blinds improve the acoustics of the room. It is also useful to have something to blackout the windows, if you need to show a video or slides.

Acoustics

What are the acoustics of the room like? You will probably find that a large auditorium will require amplification. Check out what sort of system is available.

It is vital that the room has adequate sound proofing to prevent partici-pants being disturbed by external noises. Is it near a noisy street? This may be a problem if participants need to open the windows for some fresh air.

Catering

The type and extent of the catering will be determined by the size and length of the meeting and, ultimately, your budget. Check the on site catering facilities. You may need to arrange an external caterer. Companies will provide a range of services from sandwiches to full catering.

At the very least, there needs to be something to drink. Still water is useful for members during the meeting, and tea or coffee for refreshment breaks. If money is an issue, ask members to contribute towards the cost.

Access

Is there disabled access? This includes access to toilets.

Booking the venue

Book your venue well in advance. Allow some extra time before and after the meeting. This allows you to prepare the room at the beginning, and to clear away after the meeting. Provide the organisers with the details of your requirements, and get confirmation in writing.

Pre-meeting preparation

It is good idea if the chairperson or secretary check the venue before the start of the meeting. Particular attention needs to be paid to the set-up of the room. Is there adequate seating? Are there writing surfaces? Is the temperature comfortable? Any papers and writing materials need to be distributed, and name plaques put in position.

Summary points

- Decide the date and time of your meeting.
- Select appropriate members to attend.
- Circulate all the members with an agenda. This is a statement of the purpose and content of the meeting. It will also include details of the time, date and place of the meeting.
- Send up-to-date travel details if this is appropriate.
- Include any papers members need to study before the meeting with the agenda.
- Choose a venue carefully. Think about location, facilities, type of accommodation and catering.
- Book the venue well in advance of the date of your meeting.

Checklist For Organising A Meeting

Organisation:

☐ Is the venue booked?

> *Location:*

Date/length of time booked for:............................

No. of participants:............................

Refreshments required:

☐ Coffee/tea

☐ Soft drinks

☐ Bottled water

☐ Biscuits

☐ Buffet lunch/sandwiches

☐ Full lunch

Room lay-out required:

☐ Board room

☐ Auditorium

☐ Informal

No of chairs:............................

Communication

☐ Have you circulated the minutes of the previous meeting?

☐ Has the final agenda been circulated to members?

☐ Have you included comprehensive travel details?

☐ Have you sent any papers that require reading in preparation for the meeting?

Audio-visual aids required:

☐ Whiteboard

☐ Flip chart

☐ OHP

☐ Slide projector

☐ Video playback

Organiser informed of requirements ☐

Any other equipment:...

13

Communication Roles

There are three main roles in a meeting – the chairperson, the secretary and the member. Each of these roles places different communicative demands on the individual. This section looks at each role in turn, and offers some practical advice about communication skills.

ROLE OF THE CHAIRPERSON

Obviously this is the most demanding role in a meeting. It involves skills in leadership, planning and diplomacy. Chairing your first meeting can be nerve wracking. To ensure that you perform as an effective chair, you need to prepare adequately. Your first step is planning a structure for the meeting.

Setting the agenda

The agenda helps to shape the meeting by providing a structure and focus for the group's deliberations. It is also a source of information. The members are told why they are meeting and what they will be discussing. For the chair, the agenda is an invaluable tool for keeping the group on task.

Consequently you need to give careful consideration to how you set the agenda. You will have several aims that include:

- To keep everyone interested
- To get everybody involved
- To get through the business
- To fulfil objectives.

It is customary to start the agenda with apologies for absence, minutes of the previous meeting and matters arising. The rest of the agenda will be a mixture of your ideas, suggestions from the meeting members and regular items. Think about what you want the meeting to achieve. Do you need to make progress in a certain area? Have you got any decisions to make? What actions do the members need to implement?

Once you have a list of items, place them in order of priority. Some may need urgent attention, and therefore need to be dealt with as soon as possible although, as chair, your aim is to minimise the number of emergency debates. A crisis agenda can be avoided by working out the external pressures for each item. For example, you will need to discuss a grant application several months before the closing date. This will help you deal with matters in good time.

The other thing to avoid is the reverse situation of having items on the agenda too soon. For example, there is no point in discussing an issue if vital information is unavailable. Some items will therefore need to be deferred to a later date.

Your selection of items will also be influenced by time constraints. The number you can deal with will depend upon the length of the meeting, and the content of each item. Work out how long each item will take to present, plus an estimate of the time for the subsequent discussion.

The order in which you deal with items is crucial. Put essential business items at the beginning. This avoids the problem of them being talked out by enthusiastic debates over more controversial issues. Generally items that are likely to provoke a lot of discussion are better in the middle (although it is not always easy to predict which ones are controversial). Plan one or two final items that will help the group finish on a successful note.

Of course not every item will be of interest or need the involvement of all the members. Spread out the more mundane items, and avoid grouping together items that apply to only a few members. Otherwise people will be spending large amounts of time either bored or uninvolved in the proceed-ings. Alternatively, you could place items that require just a few key people at the end of the meeting. Other members who are not needed are then free to go.

You should now have a clear outline. Make a final check that the order of the agenda is logical. For example, some items need to be discussed before you can move on to other ones. The last item to place on your agenda is a slot for any other business (AOB). Some people prefer to do without this section. However, it does allow the members to give any quick notices that have arisen since the agenda was set.

Problems arise if members use this section for bringing up controversial issues. This can be dealt with by suggesting that the member put it forward for discussion at the next meeting. If this happens on a regular basis, you may need to ask yourself if you are allowing members enough participation in setting the main agenda.

When planning your agenda remember:

- The agenda is about items now or in the future. Avoid going over past problems or mistakes.

- Variety is the spice of life. Think about the length of each item. Intersperse shorter ones amongst longer and weightier issues. Try to break up the more routine items with a few interesting ones.

- Book outside speakers either at the beginning or end of a meeting. This way there is less disruption to the meeting as a whole.

- Try to finish on a positive note.

Notification

Circulate a notice of your final agenda to members well in advance of the meeting. This may need to be several months in advance if the meeting is a large one such as an annual general meeting. Your notice will give the title and purpose of the meeting, when (date, start and finish times) and where it will take place.

Include a list of numbered agenda items. Describe these clearly using specific rather than general statements. Write them as goals or objectives, for example 'to make a decision' or 'to decide upon'. This will help members to prepare properly for the meeting.

Here is an example of an agenda:

**Heads of Departments Meeting
Agenda**

To be held at Cherry Orchard House, at 2.30.pm. on Wednesday the 5th May, 1995.

(1) Apologies for absence.

(2) Minutes of the previous meeting.

(3) Matters arising.

(4) A review of hospital transport.

(5) Preparation of a response to the plans for the new rehabilitation unit.

(6) Organisation of hospital Fete.

(7) AOB.

Finish 3.30.pm

Preparation

Like any other member you will need to read through the relevant documentation for the meeting. In addition you may also want to try to anticipate if any difficulties might arise in the meeting. Will any of the members have a hidden agenda? Are there any likely to be any personality clashes? Are some items extremely controversial? Thinking ahead in this way allows you to plan how you will cope with these different situations.

Opening the meeting

The day of the meeting has arrived. Your first task is to open the meeting. The best start is a punctual one. This means arriving on time yourself, preferably before the other members. You will then be there to welcome them as they arrive. It also means starting the meeting at the time announced on the agenda. A good motto is 'never to punish the punctual members by waiting for those who are late'.

Like any other social encounter you will start with an introduction. The way in which you introduce yourself will depend on the type of meeting and how well you know the members. Obviously you do not need to tell colleagues who you are, but in a large formal meeting you would introduce yourself and thank members for attendance.

Part of your introduction will be to remind the group of the purpose of the meeting, and if appropriate some of the meeting procedures. At this point the agenda is presented and members are asked for their agreement. Additions to the agenda may occur if an emergency item arises, but it is best to discourage last minute changes that do not allow proper preparation.

In some circumstances it may be appropriate for the members to suggest a change to the order of items, or even whether an item needs to be deferred. This can happen for a number or reasons. For example, if a key member finds that they have to leave the meeting early, they might ask for the item to be brought forward (or dealt with early on in the meeting).

After your introductions it is customary to report any apologies for absence. (This is also a good time to introduce new members to the group.) Then a check is made of the previous meeting's minutes, and any matters arising are noted. The former involves the members in identifying any inaccuracies in recording. This is not an opportunity for members to change a decision or rewrite the debate. Comments are limited to errors in factual detail, such as the misspelling of an address. Matters arising are any issues pertaining to the agenda items listed in the minutes. For example, a member may report back on their progress.

Once these routine procedures have been completed your job is to introduce the first item. Explain why it is on the agenda and provide any background information as necessary. Then start the discussion by asking members to speak to the item.

Your main role in the following discussion is to keep the group on task and ensure they achieve their targets. These targets are best elicited from the group, rather than imposed by the chair. Involving the members in setting the agenda is one way of ensuring they are included in choosing these targets. The members are then more likely to feel committed to achieving them.

Encouraging participation

Some group members find it very difficult to participate in discussion, particularly if there is a large group or they are unfamiliar with other members. Your role as chair is to encourage everyone to join in the debate. The way that you phrase questions can affect how much information members contribute to the meeting. Open questions are more likely to encourage discussion. A question like 'John, can you give us an update on in-service training?' will start the debate. A closed question like 'How much has been spent on training?' can be used later on to get specific details.

You also need to think about how you will react when members do make a contribution. The way that you respond may either encourage or discourage further comment. This is not the time to be sifting through your notes. Although members will look for acknowledgement from the group, they will particularly be seeking it from you. Use your body language to show that you are giving them your full attention. Lean forward and look at them. Use nodding and vocal encouragements such as 'mm-hmm' to show that you are listening. Remember to monitor your facial expression, as this is a strong source of feedback for the speaker. Try to keep a neutral expression. Any hint of disapproval is likely to curtail the speaker and make them think twice about making any other comments. However, be careful not to appear to be in agreement where none exists.

Some members will need more direct encouragement to express their opinions. As the chair, you need to draw them into the discussion. This can be as simple as asking for an opinion 'David, what do you think about this proposal'. (Give a general warning that you are going to ask for opinions, before you put the spotlight on one person.)

There will be some members who appear to be deliberately withholding their participation. You will need to tackle these people if the behaviour is consistent over time, as it can subtly affect the dynamics of the meeting. Do this after the meeting. A non-confrontational approach is best – something like 'I have always found your contributions valuable, but I've noticed you're not saying very much these days. Why is that?' will encourage the person to discuss the problem.

Controlling difficult members

The withdrawn member is only one example of the difficult personalities who we encounter in meetings. We have all sat through meetings where one or two people have dominated the discussion. They often have their own agenda or a particular hobby horse. It is also probably true to say that they have said all these things many times before at previous meetings. Here are some common examples of difficult members and how to deal with them:

The late comer

This does not refer to the person who occasionally turns up late. This is the persistent offender. Problems with punctuality have to be dealt with if they are occurring on a regular basis. They not only disrupt the flow of the meeting, but it will also presumably mean that the member is missing out on vital information. (People who leave the meeting early or pop in and out also come into this category.)

Excuses for this type of behaviour such as 'I was busy seeing clients' or 'I need to go and meet up with somebody' must be challenged. This can be done openly within the group. At the end of the meeting when it comes time to book the next meeting, make a point of asking the person if she will be able to make the time. This can be presented in terms of 'we would really like your input, so can we find a time you are available'. Once you have agreed on a time, check with her again. She should get the message fairly quickly.

The antagonist

This is the person who acts like Attilla the Hun. She is aggressive in both manner and approach, treating issues on a personal level, and clashing with other members. You need to make it clear to these members that this sort of behaviour is unacceptable. Never allow a personal attack to continue. Interrupt and bring the meeting back to the agenda.

The 'yes, but' person

This person dismisses every proposal out of hand. You need to deal firmly with his objections. Enlist the support of the other members in countering his negativity by asking for their opinions on the proposal.

The self-appointed representative

This person begins with 'I know I am speaking for the junior members of staff when I say…' In reality they probably do not accurately reflect the views of other people. Instead it is a strategy to allow the person to put forward (usually controversial) points, without taking the responsibility. Insist that if members have a point to make they speak for themselves only.

The dominator

This member will attempt to dominate the discussion, often interrupting other members or refusing to hand over to another speaker. In a formal meeting you will have considerable control over who talks and when they talk. On occasions you may want to use the 'through the chair' rule. This is when members have to address their comments strictly to the chair, who indicates when someone is allowed to talk. On the whole such a regimented approach is not required, and should be reserved for use with very disruptive members.

Motor mouth

This is the person who talks at length about every topic, whether they have a valid contribution to make or not. Sometimes this is due to innocent motives like wanting to make the meeting lively or keep the discussion going. Less worthy motives include a desire to control the meeting and thereby the decision making. You will on occasions have to block these members. This then gives others a chance to contribute. The way you do this is really the reverse of what you do to encourage participation. Avoid giving them any encouragement, for example through eye-contact. Use closed questions rather than open, and if necessary say you want to hear the views of other people. This can be presented in a friendly manner without being confrontational.

Remember not all meetings have members who are so awful as the examples above. Other people at the meeting will be positive in their approach, and able to make useful contributions. Examples of good meeting members include those who are:

- Positive and optimistic
- Good at thinking up ideas
- Logical and objective
- Informative
- Considered in their opinions

- ○ Analytical
- ○ Quick to identify the key issues.

Make a point of involving these people in the discussion.

Helping the group reach a decision

Meetings are about making decisions. You can help facilitate this process by clarifying issues for members and drawing together the various threads of the debate.

Use the following strategies in the meeting:

- ○ Concentrate on listening to the arguments, and avoid getting too immersed in the debate. A good chair spends more time listening than talking.
- ○ Help clarify points by asking questions or reflecting statements. For example, 'So you are saying the timing of the clinic is the problem'.
- ○ Draw members' attention to points of agreement.
- ○ Use summaries to bring together the main points of the discussion.
- ○ Highlight any gaps in information by asking questions to stimulate people's thoughts. For instance 'Do we know what the budget for non-pay was last year?'
- ○ Remind people of the agenda if they wander off the point.
- ○ Help the group to examine areas of disagreement.
- ○ If you are going to ask for a vote on a decision, summarise both the arguments for and against.

ROLE OF THE SECRETARY

Most meetings need some form of secretary. You may find yourself elected to this position, or you may have chosen to take it on out of interest. You will help the chair in preparing the agenda, and notifying the members of the date and venue. During the meeting you will need to ensure its smooth running, for example by providing spare copies of minutes for any members who have forgotten to bring a copy.

Taking the minutes

One of the key administrative duties in a meeting is taking the minutes. It is important to decide who will do this before the meeting. In an informal situation this role can be shared between members, who can take it in turns to minute the meeting. In a formal situation an official minute taker needs to be appointed. It is difficult to take the minutes and participate fully in a meeting. Therefore it is better to elect somebody who will have little involvement in the discussions. The ideal person is often the secretary. This person can then concentrate on their administrative functions.

The skills required by the two roles are also very similar. First, you need to be a good listener. Meetings can be lengthy, with detailed discussions between members, some of whom will be poor speakers who mumble or give rambling monologues. You will need to be able to extract and summarise the main points of their discussion.

Good written skills are also essential. As secretary, you will be familiar with preparing documentation for the meeting. You will also have an understanding of procedures. This will assist you in organising the information in the minutes appropriately. These need to be recorded accurately and clearly, and contain no ambiguities. If you have word processing skills you can record the minutes instantaneously using a lap-top computer.

Why do we need minutes?

Minutes are an agreed record of the discussions and resolutions of a meeting. They help remind members of what has happened at previous meetings, thereby preventing any unnecessary repetition of items. Apart from being an *aide memoire*, they are also an important check on the progress of the work of members. They document not only the decisions of a meeting, but how, when and by whom these decisions will be implemented.

Minutes are a major source of information within an organisation. Copies can be supplied to people who have not attended the meeting. For example, minutes from a meeting of heads of department can be circulated to all departmental staff.

Writing the minutes

You have been elected to take the minutes, but how do you go about it? Start by recording basic administrative details such as the date, time, and the place where the meeting is taking place. You also need to make a note of who has attended. The easiest way is to send round a piece of paper for people to write their name and occupation. The names of absent members are recorded under 'apologies'. It is customary only to include those people who have sent apologies either before the meeting or through one of the members who is present.

The style of minutes varies between meetings. The minutes of a large annual general meeting will be very different from an impromptu gathering of colleagues to discuss a new piece of equipment. However, it is possible to identify some essential elements.

The structure of your minutes is on the whole provided by the agenda. Use the number and heading from the agenda to identify each item. For example, Item 2 'Hospital transport'.

It is only necessary to record the main points of the discussion and a summary of any verbal reports. However, in practice this is a demanding task. You need to identify and note relevant information, whilst attempting to follow the next point. Some people take very full notes at the time, and summarise the information later. This is a very time consuming method. It is advisable to develop the ability to note the main points using a few words. You will improve your accuracy if you complete your final draft of the minutes as soon as possible after the meeting when your memory of events is still fresh.

On serious items you also need to make a note of any dissension amongst the members. Be careful to remain objective in your comments. Do not worry too much about who said what. Record only the main arguments against the proposal and avoid giving opinions or interpretations.

The most important thing to note in the minutes are the meeting's resolutions. These need to be recorded verbatim. Check with the chair if you are not sure how to word a particular decision.

These decisions will often involve members in taking some sort of action. It is essential that this is noted under action points, with the names of the members responsible for implementing them. Include a date for either completing the task, or reporting back on progress. It is essential to record this detail for a number of reasons. One is that it gives members the authority to act. If anyone challenges an action taken by a member, they can be referred to the minutes. Another is that it makes the member accountable to the group. The member will be expected to carry out the action as agreed. By including deadlines it also acts as a check on the progress of this work.

Your final section will be any other business. Record under this heading any items that have been raised by members since the agenda was set. Use the same format you would use for any other agenda item. End your minutes with the date of the next meeting and the proposed venue. Here is an example of minutes from a fictitious meeting:

Minutes of the **Heads of Departments Meeting** held at Cherry Orchard House, at 2.30.pm. on Friday the 5th May, 1995

Present: Dr A Brown (Unit Director)

Mrs A Nicols (Head of Physiotherapy)

Mr B Gregg (Head of Occupational Therapy)

Ms E Begley (Head of Speech Therapy)

Miss R Lough (Ward Sister)

Mr NB Hardman (Principal Social Worker)

(1) Apologies received from: D Piper (Head of Dietetics)

(2) Minutes of the meeting held on Friday 7th April 1995 were agreed as accurate.

(3) Matters arising:
Item 3 Updating equipment: Orlando Suppliers of Specialist Rehabilitation Equipment have been invited to visit the unit on 24th May at 3.00 p.m. They will be demonstrating several pieces of lifting equipment.

(4) Hospital transport: All departments have been experiencing severe delays in the arrival of out-patients using the hospital ambulance service.

Action Points: Dr Brown to write a letter of complaint to the transport manager this week.

(5) Plans for the new rehabilitation unit: Dr Brown tabled the plans for the new unit. Concern was expressed by Mrs Nichols about the distance between the pool and the patients changing room. All members felt the office space would be inadequate.

Action Points: Dr Brown will invite the architects to the next meeting.

(6) Hospital Fete: Miss R Lough reminded staff about the summer fete and invited ideas for fund raising events.

Action Points: All staff will circulate the information around their departments. Ideas to be submitted to Miss Lough by June 1st.

(7) Any other business: none

Date of the next meetings is Friday 2nd June 1995 at 2.30 p.m. Please note this will be held in Room X, first floor of the South Wing.

After the meeting

The work of the secretary continues after the meeting has finished. You will need to check your final draft of the minutes with the chair. She will also be able to advise you on whether any matters are confidential. If so, these items will need to be recorded separately from any minutes for general circulation.

Circulate minutes to all people who attended the meeting, and to those people who have sent apologies. This needs to be done as soon as possible after the meeting. Include any other relevant documents with the minutes.

It is a good idea to keep a master copy of the minutes in a ringbinder or box file. Leave this in a place that is accessible to other meeting members. This can then be used for reference.

THE MEETING MEMBER

Attending a meeting brings responsibilities. You need to be organised, prepared and able to participate actively in the meeting.

Organisation

The first thing you need to do is get yourself organised. Here is a light hearted look at the four things you need to do – record, acknowledge, organise travel and prepare. What is your usual response to receiving notification of a meeting?

(1) Recording the information:

☐ Carefully file it away at the back of your filing cabinet until you have time to deal with it.

☐ Bin it or use it as napkin for your leaky coffee cup.

☐ Immediately make a note of the date, venue and purpose of the meeting in your diary.

(2) Notifying your attendance to the chair:

☐ You send your reply slip to the chair the same day you receive your notification.

☐ You never make firm commitments.

☐ You ring the chair at 9.00 on the day of the meeting to inform her you are on your way.

(3) Checking travel details:

- ☐ You rely on last year's train time-table in the hope the times are roughly the same.

- ☐ You get up to date travel information, and check exactly how long the journey will take.

- ☐ You realise the day you are travelling, the meeting is in Birmingham, USA and not Birmingham, England.

(4) Preparation:

- ☐ You will have plenty of time to read your minutes and papers over coffee at the start of the meeting.

- ☐ You know you put them in a safe place, it's just that you are not sure where that safe place is.

- ☐ You read the agenda and papers well ahead of the meeting.

You do not need to be told which ones are the right choice! It is important to use a business-like approach to the meeting. By recording the date immediately, you avoid any problems of overlooking the meeting or getting yourself double booked. You need to decide between meetings if you find you are committed to another event. Never try to share your time, as this is disruptive to both you and the people with whom you are meeting.

It is also good manners to confirm you are attending as soon as possible. The organisers will need to know numbers for catering, seating and so on. If you are unable to attend they may even be able to re-arrange the meeting.

Preparation

You have a responsibility to be prepared for the meeting, just like the chair and the secretary. This starts with checking the agenda. Are there any items on which you want to speak? If so, you will probably need to do some background research by reading reports or other relevant documents. If you intend to make a proposal, you will certainly need to gather evidence and plan your presentation carefully.

It is also worth checking the minutes of the previous meeting. Be ready to provide an update report on any action points you have been asked to implement. It is much better to have thought about what you want to say, rather than ad-libbing in the meeting. This all takes time, so avoid leaving preparation till half hour before the meeting.

Making a contribution

If you feel unable to speak at the meeting all your hard work in preparing will have gone to waste. There are some tips in the section 'Presenting Self' on how to boost your confidence. There are also a number of things you can do during the meeting itself.

The first thing to do is to get a seat in the right position. The chair has considerable control over who speaks and when, so make sure you are seated in her eye-line. For instance, a seat opposite is better than one next to her.

Use your posture and facial expression to show that you are interested and involved in the proceedings of the meetings. Remember to lean forwards slightly. Using body language in this way will attract the attention of the chair, who is then more likely to include you in the discussion.

The way in which you establish a speaking turn will vary between different types of meetings. In a formal situation you will have to rely on the chair asking you to make a contribution. You need to concentrate on getting her attention. Once you know she is looking at you, give some sort of indication that you wish to speak. This might be leaning further forwards, raising an eye-brow or putting up your hand. She may ask you to speak immediately, or indicate your position if there are several speakers, that is whether you are second, third or whatever.

There are fewer rules regarding participation in less formal meetings. The debate is often fast moving and can become quite heated. You may find it difficult, especially if you are more reticent than others, to get a turn at speaking. However, it is important to make a contribution. Freeburn (1994) likens meetings to a team game. The successful team player gets the ball onto the field as soon as possible. In other words you need to make a contribution early in the meeting.

Think about what you are going to say. Bales (1970) found that people who tend to contribute less in meetings are more likely to use a speaking turn to acquiesce with other members. Although this sort of reinforcement is important for group cohesion, you also need to make an active contribution. Are there any facts and figures you can provide to help clarify the discussion? What is your opinion about the issue under debate? People will be interested to hear your views. Adding to the meeting in this way will also increase your credibility.

Once you know what you want to say you need to get a turn at speaking. Try to get eye-contact with the present speaker by turning towards them. This lets them know that you have something to say. Usually people will finish off their point, and hand over to you. If not, you need to interrupt them. Wait till they are at the end of a sentence and have preferably concluded a point. Deliver your point quickly and firmly. Sometimes it can help if you start by picking up on one or two words in the speaker's last sentence and incorporating these into the beginning of your message.

Present your ideas clearly and concisely. Use a firm delivery and be determined not to give way until you have finished. Any sign of hesitation will be pounced upon by more vociferous members in the group, who will see it as a chance to continue expounding their views.

The way in which you structure your sentences can also affect how people perceive your message. Avoid the following constructions which will reduce the effectiveness of your delivery:

(1) Tags: These are little phrases tagged onto the end of statements. For example, 'The policy needs refining. Doesn't it.'

(2) Disclaimers: These are statements like 'I may be wrong, but I think...' or 'This is not really my point of view, but I will tell you anyway...'

(3) Qualifiers – These are statements that moderate your argument. For example, they state the limits of when and how something can be applied. These are excellent when used in the correct place. This is after your main point not before. Never start your argument with a qualifying statement.

You can use a little bit of psychology in your approach to the meeting. For example, the group is much more likely to accept a suggestion than a straight forward proposal. An opening that starts with 'What do people think about...' is better than 'This is what needs to be done'. The group are less likely to argue with the former.

Non-verbal behaviours can also support your message. It will help if you look up rather then down at your papers. Although your main focus is the chair of the meeting, try to glance round at all the members. Using eye-contact in this way shows that you are addressing your comments to the whole group and not just making an aside.

After the meeting

You may have been allocated one or two tasks, which it will be your responsibility to implement. It is easy to forget this once the meeting has finished so try to develop some sort of system that will remind you of what you need to do. This can be as simple as an action points list on your wall.

You may also need to provide feedback for people not at the meeting. For instance, if you are representing your department on a committee, you will need to report what happened. Prepare a précis of the main points.

Action Points

Chairperson

(1) Use this checklist to evaluate your agenda:

☐ Does it state the purpose of the meeting?

☐ Does it give the date and venue for the meeting?

☐ Are the items numbered?

☐ Is each item clearly described?

☐ Do you have all the information you need for each item?

☐ Do items vary in length?

☐ Are the important business items at the beginning?

☐ Have you time-tabled speakers at the beginning or the end?

☐ Is the sequence logical?

☐ Are you starting and finishing on a positive note?

(2) Use the following checklist to evaluate your communication skills in leading a meeting. (You can ask a colleague to observe one of your meetings.)

Approximate ratio of talk by chair and talk by members chair __% members __%

☐ Used summaries to help clarify situations

☐ Asked questions if discussion became unclear

☐ Differences of opinion were elicited

☐ Provided leads to move the discussion forward

☐ Encouraged quieter members to participate

☐ Successfully blocked dominant members

☐ Adequate control of the meeting was maintained

☐ Summaries of arguments for and against a decision were provided

☐ Manner was confidant and controlled

Secretary

(1) Use this checklist to help you prepare for the meeting:

Meeting materials:

☐ Paper/notepads

☐ Handouts

☐ Pens/pencils

☐ Board markers

☐ Board eraser

☐ OHP pens (non-permanent in assorted colours)

☐ Large felt-tips

☐ Name badges

☐ Place cards

Prepared materials

☐ Prepared acetates

☐ Spare acetates

☐ Video Tapes

☐ Slides

Member

(1) Listen to how other members gain a speaking turn. Are they successful? Does the interrupted person relinquish their turn? Note in particular the responses to the following ways of attempting a speaking turn:

- Talking loudly over the other person before they have finished.
- Interrupting at the end of a sentence, but the speaker is mid-way in making a point.
- Interrupting at the end of a sentence when the speaker has finished making a point.
- Ceasing to give any listener feedback.
- Interrupting abruptly with 'Can I say something here?'
- Picking up on one or two words said by the speaker, and then continuing with their own point.
- Using non-verbal cues to indicate they want a turn, leaning forwards for example.

(2) Observe the different contributions members make. Use the following categories to help you.

- Giving information
- Seeking information
- Objecting
- Making a suggestion
- Offering an opinion
- Making a joke
- Asking for clarification
- Agreeing
- Acknowledging or praising another member
- Criticising
- Suggesting a compromise.

Summary Points

Chairperson

- The chair plans a structure for the meeting by setting an agenda. The agenda provides a focus for the group and is also a source of information.

- The chair opens the meeting by stating its purpose and presenting the agenda.

- The main role of the chair during the meeting is to keep the group on task and ensure the group achieve their stated targets.

- The chair makes sure that everyone joins in the debate by encouraging more reticent members to make a contribution. It is also the role of the chair to control more difficult members.

- Meetings are about making decisions. The chair helps this process by clarifying the issues for members and drawing together the various threads of the debate.

The secretary

- Your main duties as secretary will be organisational and administrative.

- One of the key administrative duties in a meeting is taking the minutes. This is often best done by the meeting's secretary.

- You need to be a good listener. This is essential if you are going to record the discussion accurately.

- You also need good written skills to summarise information clearly and concisely.

- Minutes are an agreed record of the discussions and resolutions of a meeting. They act as an aide-memoire and a source of information to meeting members.

- Minutes record who is present at the meeting, the main points of the discussion, decisions and who will implement these decisions.

Meeting member

- ◦ Attending meetings requires you to be organised, prepared and able to participate actively.

- ◦ Check the agenda well before the meeting and prepare any points you want to make to the other members.

- ◦ Read any relevant material that has been sent to you.

- ◦ It is important that you make a contribution in the meeting, and that you do this as soon as possible.

- ◦ Where you sit will affect your chances of being able to establish a speaking turn. Make sure you get a seat in the eye-line of the chair.

- ◦ Present your ideas clearly and concisely using a firm tone of voice.

- ◦ Support your message non-verbally.

14

Presenting Self

You may feel that meetings are not important enough to worry about how you present yourself. In fact they can have a considerable impact on your credibility. The manner in which you behave and the quality of your contributions are ways of getting yourself noticed by senior managers. Think about the meetings that you attend. How much contact do you have with these staff apart from meetings? The meeting may be the only opportunity they get to view your performance. It is up to you whether the attention you attract is positive or negative.

Motivation

Meetings are often boring, unproductive, hostile or apathetic. This is the reason that many people try to avoid them altogether. To start changing this scenario, you first need to develop a positive attitude. Think about the benefits that meetings provide. Here are just a few examples:

- You have the chance to find out what is going on in both your department and elsewhere in the organisation.

- You are able to meet colleagues with whom you have little contact during the normal course of events. Without this contact it is easy to become isolated.

- Meetings are a way of sharing a task. You can elicit support for a problem you are facing, or use the group's ideas to progress a project.

- Meetings are about making decisions. By attending a meeting you will have the opportunity to become involved in the decision making process.

- Managers use meetings to disseminate information to their staff. This is often about their expectations of staff performance. It is important that you are aware of these expectations, and are able to give feedback to managers.

○ Meetings are about communication. This is not just about management giving information to staff. Members can use meetings to communicate to other staff and to management itself. This might be a report to update the members on your progress on a particular project, or to provide some information about a new idea or piece of equipment.

○ Finally, meetings are an opportunity to demonstrate your talents. These might be leadership skills, initiative or diplomacy.

Presenting yourself

You need to think about how you present to other people. The things that you do are just as important as what you say. Remember:

Be punctual

Famous film stars will arrive late to make an impression. Late comers disrupt events, and therefore attract everybody's attention. This is fine for celebrities, but not for more ordinary folk. Arriving late for a meeting is distracting, and you will also miss out on some of the discussion.

Be organised

Make sure you are organised. Bring all the relevant papers including the agenda and minutes from the previous meeting. Show everybody you are ready by placing them in order on the meeting's table.

Be conscious of your image

Your appearance does matter. This is not about power dressing. It is about choosing the right clothing for the occasion. Meetings are a bit like parties. They are either formal or informal. You will stand out like a sore thumb if you dress casually at a formal event. So match your outfit to the occasion. (There is some advice about formal dressing in the chapter on *Recruitment Interviews.*)

Be positive

Think of things you can contribute to the meeting. Is there an item on the agenda about which you can provide some background information? Can you offer a solution to another member's problem?

Be enthusiastic and interested

Use your body language to show that you are interested in the meeting. Remember this applies to how you enter the room, your posture during the meeting and how you act at refreshment breaks.

Here are some examples of behaviours to avoid at a meeting. These are all based on actual events and real people!

- Falling asleep
- Knitting
- Writing memos, letters
- Reading magazines
- Staring dreamily out of the window
- Cutting off split ends from strands of hair
- Extensive doodling
- Drawing cartoons of other members.

Be confident

Confidence is essential, whether you are about to chair your first meeting, or you just want to participate more actively. Developing the self assurance you need will take time. It is not something that you switch on and off at the start and finish of a meeting. Learning to appreciate your talents and skills is an important part of this process. Heylin (1991) suggests keeping what she terms as an 'ego file'. You fill the file with evidence of previous achievements. These can vary from a cycling proficiency certificate to a special award. A quick look through the file will help build up your self esteem.

Be an active member

Get the most out of your meeting. Ask questions if you are unsure, particularly if you have to implement any action points; and take notes to help you remember key points. Think about how you can put into practice what you have learnt from the meeting.

Be a good listener

Develop active listening. Set yourself a series of questions for the meeting. For example: What relevance is this information to me? How does it affect other people? What is the importance of this information to the subject under discussion?

Be sensitive to the views of other people – It is sometimes difficult to accept the views or opinions of people with whom we may disagree. Part of successful debate and discussion in a meeting is being able to accept that the people have the right to express their views.

Summary Points

- Meetings are an opportunity to present a positive image to senior staff.

- Attending a well-managed meeting offers many benefits. Meetings are a forum for communication between staff and management, and an opportunity for individuals to participate in decision making and problem solving.

- Presenting yourself effectively involves thinking about how you behave as well as what you say.

- It is important to be punctual, organised, and to have the appropriate attitude to other people.

Action Points

(1) Think about the different meetings that you attend. List the benefits you get from attending these meetings. What information would you miss if you failed to attend? What contributions did you make at your last meeting?

(2) You may be feeling nervous about a particular meeting. Is it your first professional meeting since qualifying? Are you daunted by the prospect of a large, formal meeting? Is this the first time you have chaired a meeting?

Try these tips to help you calm your nerves:

- Make sure you allow plenty of time to travel to the meeting. Arrive early so that you are able to spend five or ten minutes relaxing and settling yourself into your seat.

- Try some 'in your seat relaxation':
  - Sit comfortably with your shoulders relaxed. Avoid slouching.
  - Give your toes a wiggle to get rid of any tension. (I have chosen 'toes' because they are hidden away. No one will know what you are doing.)
  - Slow down your breathing. (There are some useful exercises on breathing in the *Effective Use of Voice* chapter.)
  - Give yourself something to think about. Re-read your minutes, or write out a list of questions you have about the agenda.

Meeting Skills in Context
Business Meetings

Business meeting is a term often used to refer to the semi-informal staff meetings held in most departments on a regular basis. These meetings help managers and staff deal with matters that arise on a regular basis. They are usually chaired by the head of the department or the service manager, and are formally recorded using the standard format of minutes.

Why do you need to have business meetings?

Meetings provide a channel for communication between staff and management (Gratus 1990). Information can be quickly distributed to a large number of people. To mail the same number of staff would be time consuming, with any queries having to be dealt with on an individual basis. Giving information during a meeting also allows staff the opportunity to clarify points immediately with their manager. In responding to one question she may well have provided answers to similar queries from several other staff.

This communication channel is two-way. Staff are able to give comments and suggestions to the management. Consulting staff in this way improves decision making, and increases staff commitment to the organisation's plans. Even if staff disagree they will have had the chance to let off steam about the issue. The meeting acting as a tension breaker.

Meetings are also used by managers to control the flow of work (The 3-M Meeting Management Team). Decisions are made about what needs to happen and who will carry out the work. Minutes are a record of these decisions, and a check can be made on the progress of this work by reviewing previous action points.

Although meetings are not viewed as social occasions, they do satisfy the need people have to come together as a group. Scheduling a break in the meeting allows time for members to have a chat and exchange news. Coming together as a group is also a way of helping staff to develop a sense of belonging, both to the department and to the overall organisation. This is particularly important for those professionals who spend a large amount of time working alone.

What is the best size for a meeting?

The number of meetings that people are required to attend is increasing. They take up valuable time and resources, and it is therefore essential that they are worth the effort for the individual. Sometimes meetings become a habit, something that always happens on a Wednesday afternoon. It is well worth reviewing the purpose of regular meetings, and in particular their membership. Are people selected by what they can contribute, or are they invited as a matter of course? Do you need to have a large meeting, or will a smaller group of people suffice? Only select people who really need to be there. Remember you can often improve the quality of members' participation by decreasing the number of meetings they have to attend.

In a small meeting of ten or fewer people, it is easier for members get to know each other, and therefore the atmosphere tends to be more relaxed. This informality encourages shyer members to participate. The fewer numbers also mean that organisation is simpler, and meetings can be set up at short notice to deal with emergencies.

There are some disadvantages to small groups. The smaller membership means that it is difficult to ensure that members are representative. This may make some people feel they are excluded from the decision making process. The other problem is that the lack of formality encourages the members to view it purely as a social get together.

A larger meeting has the advantage that the membership is more likely to represent a wider range of interests. However, the increased number means that there is less time for individuals to contribute. Some members may also be inhibited from speaking out in front of such a large group of people. This can often result in a few members dominating the meeting.

Large meetings also take much more organisation. A suitable venue needs to be found, and arranging a date is difficult with so many different people to accommodate. This means that notification needs to be sent out well before the actual date of the meeting.

How successful was your meeting?

If you are chairing a meeting, it is important you evaluate its effectiveness. Use the 'Meetings Checklist' to judge if your meeting was successful. Write down the reasons if something failed to happen. For example, members were unprepared because they received vital papers only hours before the meeting.

Give out the 'Members Checklist' to get feedback from your meeting members. Do their comments agree with your evaluation? These checklists will help you improve your meetings skills.

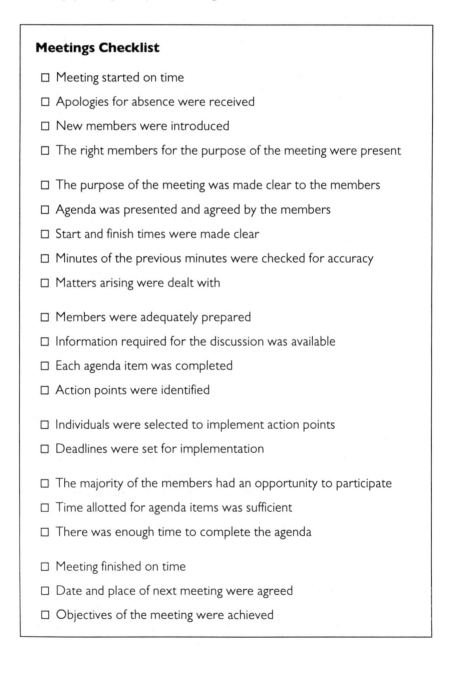

Meetings Checklist

☐ Meeting started on time

☐ Apologies for absence were received

☐ New members were introduced

☐ The right members for the purpose of the meeting were present

☐ The purpose of the meeting was made clear to the members

☐ Agenda was presented and agreed by the members

☐ Start and finish times were made clear

☐ Minutes of the previous minutes were checked for accuracy

☐ Matters arising were dealt with

☐ Members were adequately prepared

☐ Information required for the discussion was available

☐ Each agenda item was completed

☐ Action points were identified

☐ Individuals were selected to implement action points

☐ Deadlines were set for implementation

☐ The majority of the members had an opportunity to participate

☐ Time allotted for agenda items was sufficient

☐ There was enough time to complete the agenda

☐ Meeting finished on time

☐ Date and place of next meeting were agreed

☐ Objectives of the meeting were achieved

Member's Checklist

Date:
Meeting:

Please circle your response to the following questions, and write comments where requested. This information will be used to improve the quality of future meetings.

- Did you have enough notification of the meeting?   YES/NO
- Did you receive all the relevant papers?   YES/NO
- Were these received with adequate time to read and
  prepare for the meeting?   YES/NO
- Were you clear about what was expected of you in
  the meeting?   YES/NO
- Was the meeting scheduled at a convenient time for you? YES/NO
  If not, why not?

- Was the location of the meeting convenient for you?   YES/NO
  If not, why not?

- Did the meeting start on time?   YES/NO
- Was the purpose of the meeting made clear to you?   YES/NO
- Were you clear about your role in the meeting?   YES/NO
- Were the meeting's procedures made clear?   YES/NO
- Did you agree to the agenda?   YES/NO
- Were there any items you thought needed to be
  included on the agenda?
- Did you get a chance to contribute?   YES/NO
- Were you able to express your feelings?   YES/NO
- Did you feel that one or two people dominated the
  discussion?   YES/NO
- Did you feel the chair had adequate control of the
  meeting?   YES/NO
- Was the final decision 'owned' by the whole group?   YES/NO
- Did you find the meeting useful?   YES/NO
  If not, what could have been done to make it more
  helpful?

Summary Points

- Business meeting is a term often used to refer to the semi-informal staff meetings held in most departments on a regular basis.

- These meetings are a two way channel of communication between staff and management. They are also a way for management to control the flow of work within a department.

- Managers need to regularly review the membership of these meetings. A smaller meeting with key staff may be more productive.

- There are advantages to small meetings, that include easier preparation and increased participation.

- It is important to evaluate each meeting.

Meetings Skills in Context
Multi-Disciplinary Teams

Multi-disciplinary teams have always existed in the health service. This tradition continues, but the composition of these teams and the way in which they are managed has altered. These changes relate to new styles of management and alternative approaches to health care provision. The old hierarchical style is being replaced by one that encourages all staff to participate in decision making.

What is a multi-disciplinary team?

A team consists of a group of people working together towards a common objective. In the health service these teams are often multi-disciplinary, in that they bring together representatives from various disciplines. The client centred team is the most common, with the focus firmly on the care and management of the client. Members of the team are selected according to their functional relationship to the client. A child development team is one example of a multi-disciplinary team, where paediatricians, therapists and psychologists work together to enhance the care and management of children with special needs.

What are the rewards of team working?

The best health care evolves from effective team work. It provides an opportunity for staff to share information and plan a cohesive and holistic approach to the management of the client. The perspectives provided by the various disciplines also helps to improve the quality of decision making.

Individuals benefit from the supportive atmosphere of the team, where members are able to motivate each other in sometimes very difficult situations. They also gain valuable experience of team work. These are skills that employers, now more than ever, value as an essential criterion for most job specifications.

Team building

The team meeting is central to the idea of multi-disciplinary work. The members come together to exchange information, problem solve and make decisions about individual clients. People learn how to work with each other within these meetings. All teams go through a similar learning process. There are four main stages:

(1) Exploration

(2) Focusing

(3) Gelling

(4) Achievement

(1) Exploration

The first thing team members need to do is get to know each other. Members will be asking themselves questions like:

- Why is he on the team?
- Where does she work?
- What is his level of experience?
- What are her particular interests?
- Has he been on a team before?

The action points at the end of the section give some structured exercises to help team members get to know each other, and learn what individuals can offer the team. It is also important that the team spends some time together informally, even if this is just a ten minute coffee break.

(2) Focusing

At this stage the members turn their attention to the group as a whole. They start to focus on the purpose of the team. Why has it been set up? What are its functions? The team members may have a general idea of the objectives of the team. These need to be refined into a series of specific sub-goals. It is important that these goals are shared and understood by all the team.

Along with establishing the purpose of the team, the group also need to be aware of their boundaries. For one thing they must understand the limits of their authority. How does the team fit into the overall organisational structure? What type of decisions are they allowed to take? Who are the people that have to abide by these decisions? In a similar way they also need to be aware of the extent of their responsibilities.

(3) Gelling

An effective team is one where there is an atmosphere of trust and mutual respect. Members feel free to express views and opinions openly in the group without fear of ridicule or rejection. This is not something that just happens. It needs to be nurtured carefully by the group.

(4) Achievement

A point is reached in the development of the team when all the members have sorted out their respective roles, and are working towards a common goal. The team functions as a whole, rather than a group of individuals. This is the stage when the team is most likely to achieve the best results.

Teams are not static. They need to respond to external factors that affect working practice, such as new legislation or research. Pressure is also created when staff change within the team. The departure of a few key members can significantly alter the dynamics of the group. The team may need to start the whole development process again. This is a natural characteristic of team work, which helps to keep the group dynamic.

Leading a team

Teams need a leader. This is a person who can take an overview of the proceedings and act as a focus for the group. In some circumstances it is appropriate to rotate the team leader. In other situations one person may be elected or appointed to the position. This applies particularly when the leader may have to take overall clinical responsibility for the team's decisions. In this case it would be a senior member of staff.

In addition to a clinical role, the leader also has an administrative function. She can guide the group in making decisions about how to organise the team. The sorts of questions the members need to consider include:

- How will members know what is expected of them?
- How will the group know who is doing what?
- How will individuals give feedback to the group?
- Will the connection between the actions of the different members be made clear?

These are all questions that concern interaction within the group. Procedures for team meetings must address these issues. Communication systems need to be open and involve all the members regardless of their seniority in the group.

Any communication system needs to include a plan for how the team communicates with the client, family and other outside agencies. The size of a multi-disciplinary team can be daunting for the individual who is the focus of their care. For instance, imagine the feelings of a parent entering a room full of professionals to discuss the diagnosis of her child. It is often appropriate to appoint a key person who acts as the main liaison point for the client and family.

Appointing a key person for a client may be one of the tasks of a team meeting. Chairing such meetings is similar to chairing any other type of meeting. The leader is there to facilitate discussion and make sure that all relevant information has been provided. For example, if a member has concentrated on the difficulties a client is having, the chair may want to draw out some information on the client's achievements, so that a balanced view is obtained.

A large part of team meetings is decision making. The leader can help the group settle a number of issues. What decisions need to be taken? Who makes them? Is the whole team involved? Does the chair have the final say? This will very much depend on the role of the chair. If she has overall clinical responsibility then decisions will ultimate rest with her.

Avoiding conflict

A multi-disciplinary team by definition offers a variety of perspectives, which may sometimes lead to contradictory views. However, this is a necessary part of joint assessment and management of clients. Through discussing these different opinions comes a greater understanding of the needs of the client and how these can best be met. Therefore some disagreement is to be expected in team working. It is when these differences turn into confusion and misunderstandings that conflict arises.

It is useful to examine how and why this sort of conflict occurs within teams, so that you can plan how to deal with it. Here are some common causes:

'Why am I here?' – Roles are not clearly defined, so that the team member is unsure of why they are in the team. This uncertainty is transmitted to other members who will question the individual's contribution to the team – *'Why is she here?'*.

'What's the point of all this?' – The members are unsure why there is a team. They lack a sense of purpose.

'This isn't what we are supposed to be doing' – This happens when the team has failed to agree on the purpose of the team. Each member has a very different idea of what they think are the team goals.

'I thought you were meant to be doing this' – Members need to be clear about their responsibilities. Otherwise confusion arises over who is doing what. In some cases this may lead to a duplication or cross over of functions, the complaint then being *'That's my job'.*

'I thought that had already been done.' 'No, I'm waiting for you' – Problems arise if members have not sorted out when and how things are going to happen.

'This is not the way we run things in our department' – There has been no agreement on how the team is organised and run. Each person has their own idea of procedures for use in the team.

'I don't want to upset anyone' – It sometimes happens that some team members become more concerned about how people are feeling than about the stated goals of the team. The idea is that the 'team' has to be protected at all costs.

The way that the team is structured and organised is a significant factor in reducing the type of conflict described above. Here are some guidelines:

- Make sure that roles are clearly defined, and that both all the individuals and the group understand what this means.
- Members must agree on the aims of the team. Goals need to be stated explicitly in writing to avoid any misunderstanding.
- Areas of responsibility and role boundaries need to be clearly described.
- The team need to discuss and set up processes for the implementation of tasks. This would include identifying who carries out actions, and when these will be completed.
- Teams need to have a structure and rules that determine how they operate. Each individual will be familiar with the systems used in their department. However, there can only be one system for the team. This means the team must select a way of organising itself, and be committed to this approach even if it differs from their usual experience. Obtaining agreement amongst the members is

more important than establishing a particular set of procedures. Some compromise is inevitable.

Participating in a team

The responsibilities of the team member are distinct from those created by the autonomy of working alone. The differences can be illustrated by using the analogy of horses pulling a stage coach. There are always several horses pulling together in the same direction. Picture what will happen to the coach if some of the horses started dashing off in opposite directions, or one horse decided he was going to race ahead of the others. Similarly the team member has a responsibility to adhere to the team's purpose, and work with and not against other people.

Action Points

Try this exercise with a partner from your multi-disciplinary team. It is one way of sharing and finding out information about your colleagues.

(1) It starts with each person discussing their objectives concerning a specific client. (See the example in Figure 3.1. of the objectives of a speech therapist and specialist health visitor with an infant who has recently been diagnosed as deaf).

Aims of the speech therapist

- ◦ to assess communication skills
- ◦ to advise on communication strategies
- ◦ to offer support to the family

Aims of the health visitor

- ◦ to offer support and counselling to the family
- ◦ to provide the family with appropriate information
- ◦ to identify needs within the family and liaise with other professionals as appropriate

Figure 3.1 Example of the joint objectives of a speech therapist and a specialist health visitor

---

(2) Next, each person describes the different areas of their expertise, that they would need to draw upon to meet these aims. For example, to meet the objective 'to offer support and counselling' you would need counselling skills.

Compare your responses with your partner. Some of your areas of expertise will be shared. Other areas will require the special skills of one or the other. Draw up a diagram to represent your areas of expertise like the one in Figure 3.2. Write your specialist areas under your title, and any shared areas in the middle. If one of you has a greater knowledge in a shared area, place it more towards the relevant side. You can see in Figure 3.2. that both the professionals share a knowledge of hearing loss, but the speech therapist has a more specialist understanding.

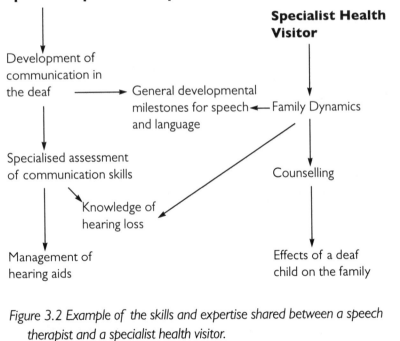

Figure 3.2 Example of the skills and expertise shared between a speech therapist and a specialist health visitor.

(3) Each person can now discuss their management of the case in the same way as their expertise. As above, areas where they are likely to be jointly involved are placed in the middle. (See Figure 3.3.)

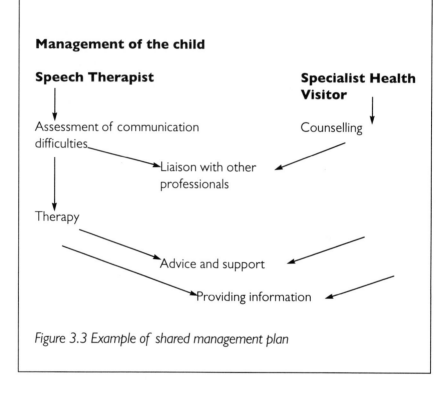

Management of the child

Figure 3.3 Example of shared management plan

This exercise will give you a greater understanding of what your partner can contribute to the team. It also helps to identify areas where your skills, and therefore your management of the client will cross over. You can then concentrate your efforts on how you are going to work together.

Checklist for a Successful Multidisciplinary Team

What makes a team work? A successful team has a number of different characteristics.

Use this checklist to evaluate your team:

☐ The team has a clear set of goals

☐ Each member understands their role within the team

☐ Members understand each other's role within the team

☐ The team has a clear purpose, which has been agreed by all members

☐ The team is able to recognise the boundaries of its authority

☐ The team is able to recognise the boundaries of its responsibilities

☐ There is an open system of communication

☐ There is an atmosphere of trust

☐ Contributions from all members are valued

☐ All members participate in the decision making

☐ Members are committed to the team and its decisions

☐ There are appropriate structures and procedures for running team meetings

☐ Conflict is managed openly within the team

Summary Points

- ○ Multi-disciplinary teams have always been integral to the health care of the client. Recent changes in management styles and approaches to health care provision have affected the composition and structure of these teams.

- ○ Most multi-disciplinary teams in the health setting are client centred. They involve representatives from the different disciplines who have a functional role with the client.

- ○ It provides an opportunity for staff to share information and plan a cohesive and holistic approach to the management of the client. The perspectives provided by the various disciplines also helps to improve the quality of decision making. Members themselves benefit from the supportive atmosphere of the team, and are able to motivate each other in sometimes very difficult situations.

- ○ Teams go through several stages of development that involve team members getting to know each other and establishing their roles within the goals of the overall team.

- ○ The nature of team work means that some disagreement is inevitable. Problem solving and decision making are improved by examining alternative perspectives.

- ○ Good structure and organisation helps to avoid conflict.

Meetings Skills in Context
Case Conferences

A case conference is a meeting called to review the management of a specific client. Its membership consists of all the professionals actively involved with the client. This includes health and non-health staff. For instance, social services and education are often involved in the case conference of a child.

Case conferences are called for a variety of reasons. These include the review of a recent assessment or the evaluation of any changes in circumstances. Sometimes the conference is part of a regular review. Not all clients will have or need a full-blown case conference. It depends on the individual client and their needs in terms of management.

Participating in a case conference for the first time can be daunting. They usually involve large groups of people, and procedures can be fairly formal. There are also emotional pressures, particularly in cases of child abuse. For this reason it is a good idea to prepare what you want to say before the conference. You need to be succinct, as there will be lots of people wanting to say things in a relatively short amount of time.

Your verbal report to the conference needs to be a summary of the main points. This should include:

- A brief outline of your role with client
- Your view of the current situation with the client
- Your anticipated role with the client in the future
- Your recommendations.

State your points clearly and without ambiguity.

Make your report as factual and informative as possible. Always back up your comments with specific examples. For example, 'I am not satisfied that Mr Buree can cope at home alone, because he is unable to manage stairs on his own. His flat is on the fourth floor, and there is no lift.'

Sometimes you may find yourself interrupted by the chair of the meeting, who is eager to get through the agenda as quickly as possible. To counteract this, introduce your report by stating what you intend to cover. For example, 'I would like to make three points' or 'I would like to discuss Tony's recent assessment, and then my recommendations arising from this evaluation.' This makes it clear to everybody where you are in giving your report.

Communicating in a case conference is not just about reporting information. You will also need to participate in decision making at the end of the meeting. To do this you need to have all the facts. Listen to what other people are saying. Does it confirm or contradict what you are saying? Does it add to your knowledge of the client? Do not be afraid to ask questions if you are unclear on any points.

Summary Points

- A case conference is a meeting called to review the management of a specific client. Its membership consists of all the professionals actively involved with the client.

- You will be expected to give an oral report about your client. Prepare this before the meeting.

- Your report needs to be a summary of your assessment and management of the case.

Meetings Skills in Context
Committees

This section tells you all about committees, and how to get the best out of them.

What is a Committee?
A committee is a group of people 'elected or appointed to perform specified functions' (Locke 1980, p.5). The duties of these members are mainly performed through the committee meeting.

How does a committee work?
All committees have some sort of constitution. This is a formal description of the rules or procedures by which the work of the committee is organised and managed. It will specify the following:

- The composition of the committee (chair, secretary, treasurer, number of other members)
- The roles and duties of the members
- The purpose and scope of the committee's work (this is also known as the 'terms of reference')
- The process for selecting officers such as the chair and so on
- The process of decision making
- The rules governing how meetings are arranged and conducted.

What do committees do?
Committees are always part of a larger organisation like a trade union, health trust or professional body. One reason for their establishment is to help disseminate decision making. Many committees have delegated powers to

make resolutions and take actions on behalf of the parent organisation. This power to make and implement decisions is a distinguishing feature of committees, although they are ultimately responsible to their parent organisation.

The other major function of committees is to provide the organisation with advice. A committee may be set up with this single purpose in mind, members being selected on the basis of their knowledge, skills or experience in a particular area. The role of a sub committee is to make recommendations to the parent organisation or to other committees; they do not have the powers to make decisions or take actions.

Why do we have committees?

Committees allow tasks to be shared amongst a number of people. The work of a large organisation can be enormous – far too much to be dealt with by a small number of senior staff. Committees are given the authority to carry out some of this work. As a result the burden of decision making is removed from a few individuals and spread amongst a group.

This idea of group responsibility is the foundation block of committee work. Members have what is known as collective responsibility. They function as one. Decisions belong to the committee as a whole and not to one or two individuals. This means that members are committed to the final resolution even if they voted against it.

There are other good reasons for having committees. A group of people are better able to represent the views of a variety of interests and opinions. This is why even relatively small groups like the local cricket club will have a committee. This way the views of all the club members can be represented. A committee is also more likely to have a range of knowledge, skills and experience.

What are the different types of committee?

There are several different types of committee.

Standing committee

This type of committee meets on a regular and permanent basis. It deals with a specified set of matters as and when they arise. Standing committees can be either executive or advisory.

Executive committee

The purpose of this type of committee is decision making. An executive committee has the final say over any decisions made by sub committees.

Advisory committee

Unlike the executive committee, this group only provides advice. They are not directly responsible for any decision taking. The usual procedure is for the committee to detail their proposals in a report to the relevant body.

Sub committee

Executive and advisory committees will often share their work out amongst a series of smaller sub committees. For example, in a professional body there may be sub committees to deal with finance, professional issues and academic matters. They report directly to the larger committee.

Ad hoc or special committee

Occasionally a committee will be set up to carry out a specific task that is short term in nature. These are also known as working parties.

Joint committee

These types of committee usually have representatives of two or more contrasting interests. For example a joint staff side committee might have representations from the management on one side, and representatives of the staff group on the other.

Chairing a committee meeting

Chairing a committee meeting is similar to chairing other meetings. However, you do need to be familiar with the constitution of the committee. One of your roles is to see that members adhere to the rules and procedures laid down in the constitution. Failure to follow these rules will compromise the legitimacy of the committee's decisions.

The constitution is also your ally in ensuring that fair debate and discussion take place. Use it to make sure that all sides have an opportunity to express their views. For instance, one basic rule is that the meeting has a quorum. This is the minimum number of people required for a meeting to be able to conduct its business. Without a quorum there is a danger that the members who are present will be unrepresentative.

As the chair you may also be involved in selecting committee members. Use the following checklist to help you to decide:

Do they have:

- ☐ Knowledge relevant to the committee's work
- ☐ Skills relevant to the committee's work
- ☐ Experience relevant to the committee's work
- ☐ Experience of committee work.

Are they good at:

- ☐ Listening
- ☐ Presenting ideas clearly
- ☐ Co-operating with other people
- ☐ Generating ideas or alternative solutions
- ☐ Making decisions
- ☐ Encouraging others
- ☐ Examining issues logically
- ☐ Analysing and evaluating ideas
- ☐ Encouraging a friendly atmosphere.

Are they:

- ☐ Outgoing and extrovert
- ☐ Quiet but thoughtful
- ☐ Caring about other members
- ☐ Energetic and vigorous in their approach.

These are just a few of the qualities you may want to consider when selecting a member. They do not represent the ideal person, as it is impossible for one person to have all of these characteristics. In fact some of them conflict with each other – the extrovert versus the quiet thoughtful person for example. These differences reflect the need for committees to have a varied member-ship.

When selecting your new member you need to take into account the characteristics of the present committee. Will the prospective member fit in? Will he help to maintain the balance between opposing interests?

Participating in a committee

The first thing to be clear about is why you are on the committee. If you have been sent as a delegate you will usually be firmly restrained in what you say and do (Anstey 1962) (although this is easily forgotten in the heat of a fierce debate). In particular you will be given instructions on how to vote on the various issues. You are there to present the views of the body you represent. For example, you may be sent as a delegate by your local branch at the regional union meeting. You will need to establish exactly what your organisation, department or association want you to say and do. After the committee meeting you will need to give some form of feedback, either orally or in writing to the body you represent.

You are more likely to find yourself as a representative. You will have much more freedom to act, compared with the delegate. However, you still need to refer back to your group in a similar way to the delegate.

As a new member you will probably need an introduction to 'committee speak'. There are numerous terms and phrases used to refer to committee procedures. Here are a few of them:

Motion: Proposals for consideration by the committee are known as motions.

Proposer: A motion needs to have someone to put it forward to the committee. This person is known as the proposer.

Amendment: This is a change to the original motion.

Point of order: This is a way of expressing that a rule or procedure has not been followed correctly.

Mandate: An order or command that you have to obey.

Standing orders: These are the rules that regulate precisely how a committee meeting is run.

Many committees are run on a semi-formal basis with a clear structure for debate. The chair is there to make sure that all the members have a fair chance to put their point of view. This makes it easier for members to participate. If you wish to speak, get the chair's attention by leaning forward or even raising your hand. Remember to be succinct as there is only a limited time for people to speak on each point.

If you wish to raise an issue you will need to put forward a motion to the chair. This will placed on the agenda of the appropriate meeting. Be prepared to speak to the committee about your proposal when it is called.

Five good reasons for being on a committee

If you need persuading to join a committee, consider the following positive points about being a member.

(1) You have a chance to influence decisions

(2) There is an opportunity to meet a variety of people

(3) You will gain experience of debate and discussion

(4) Your membership will earn you prestige and increase your credibility

(5) You will be able to effect changes in subjects or issues in which you are interested.

Action Points

(1) Find out about the committee members. Why are they on the committee?

(2) If you have a predecessor, ask their advice. They will be able to give you insider information on personalities, group dynamics and so on.

(3) Establish why you have been chosen to be a member of the committee. People are members of a committee for a variety of reasons. Which of the following apply to you?

Your position – Participation in the committee is part of the duties and responsibilities of your post.

Your status – You have been selected either because it would be rude not to include you, or in the hope your presence will give the committee prestige. Your skills and knowledge.

Your special interests – Do you have a particular interest in the subject matter of the committee? Are you concerned with the issues dealt with by the committee's parent organisation? For example, if the organisation is a voluntary association.

You find it difficult to say no – Are you there out of a sense of duty?

(4) What are your roles and responsibilities as a committee member?

Summary Points

- A committee is a group of people who are elected or appointed to carry out set duties. These are performed through the committee meeting.

- All committees have a constitution that describes the rules or procedures governing the work of the committee. The constitution provides a framework that enables a democratic debate.

- Committees have two main functions – decision making and advisory.

- The work of a large organisation can be spread out among a number of different committees. This enables the views of a wider group of people to be enlisted.

- It is important that the chair of a committee fully understands the constitution of that committee. Failure to adhere to these rules can result in decisions being invalidated.

- The main role of the chair is to ensure that a fair discussion takes place.

- Committees need to have a variety of members who are able to contribute in different ways.

- Members need to be clear about why they are on the committee and who they are representing.

- The rules and procedures make it easy for members to participate in discussions. Any proposals need to be notified to the chair, who will place them on the agenda as motions for debate.

Meetings Skills in Context
Working Parties

What is a working party?

A working party is a special kind of committee, which is also sometimes known as an *ad hoc* or special committee. These are set up to look at a particular problem, issue or task. They usually operate within a limited time period, disbanding once their purpose has been fulfilled.

If you want some experience of committee work this is probably a good choice, as it is a short term commitment. However, it is likely to involve some intensive work during the period of its existence. You will probably have work in addition to attending the meetings, which will be more frequent than other committees.

Membership

Working parties are set up to bring together people with expertise relevant to the topic under discussion. Members are selected on the basis of their skills, knowledge or experience. This ensures that the group are able to achieve an adequate understanding of the issues.

Besides background knowledge, members need to be able to think creatively. They must generate ideas, which are practicable and easily implemented. In developing these ideas the group will need to go through a process of problem solving.

Problem-solving by a working party

The aim of a working party is to come up with a solution or a set of solutions to a problem or issue that needs resolving. This is achieved by working through a number of stages. These are:

(1) Identification

The first step is identify and describe the problem. The group are then able to concentrate on the second stage of fact-finding.

(2) Investigation

Initially the group will spend a significant amount of time, gathering and discussing pertinent information. This might be facts, figures, views or opinions.

(3) Evaluation

Once the group feel they have enough data, they can start to consider various options as a solution. This is the stage when members will be contributing ideas.

(4) Decision making

The final stage is to choose the best solution to the problem. The working party are then able to make their recommendations. These might be in the form of a policy document, a report or a series of recommendations.

Participating in a working party

One advantage of participating in a working party is that it helps get you noticed within your profession and by your employers. It is therefore important to present yourself in the best way.

Follow these guidelines:

- Prepare thoroughly. Your contribution starts before the first meeting. Read any background information you think will be relevant. It is especially important to read any material sent to you by the chair.

- Working parties consist of a mixture of people representing all sorts of different backgrounds and experiences. Be aware of any bias you might have towards any members. Everybody is guilty of some prejudice. This might be about someone's age, the way they dress or their accent. Remember bias works both ways. A young person may dismiss comments from an older person as out of date. The older person may reject the idea of a young 'inexperienced' member being able to make a valuable contribution.

- Listen to what other people have to say. Do not immediately dismiss or oppose proposals that differ from your own. The final solution will be probably be a compromise.

- Make sure you have thought through your proposal before suggesting it to the group.

- Present your ideas clearly by stating one point at a time. Choosing an appropriate moment to introduce your idea to the group is also important. Avoid times when the group's concentration will be low. For instance, starting just before the tea-break is not a good time.

- Be prepared to make an active contribution, even if this means having to do some homework.

Summary Points

- A working party is a special kind of committee set up on a short term basis to look at a specific problem or issue.

- The short term commitment means they are ideal for gaining experience.

- Members need to have relevant expertise and good problem solving skills.

- Problem solving involves a number of stages that include identifying the problem, gathering information and generating solutions.

- The main qualities required to participate in a working party are good listening skills, cooperative nature and the ability to present ideas clearly.

PART FOUR

Presentation Skills

16 Preparation

17 Effective Use of Voice

18 Delivering Content

19 Establishing Rapport with the Audience

20 Using Non-Verbal Communication

21 Effective Use of Audio Visual Aids

22 Presentation Skills in Context
  22.1 Client/Carer Workshops
  22.2 Presentations to Other Professionals
  22.3 Lectures
  22.4 Selling your Service
  22.5 Presenting your Research

Presentation Skills

The main role of the health professional has always been as a provider of health care. However, in the modern health service they are also required to be educators, managers, researchers, negotiators and even salespeople. These roles often involve making presentations to clients, carers, colleagues and other professionals. A presentation can be defined as a medium for conveying a message or several messages to a group of people. There may be a single speaker or several if the presentation is a team effort.

The aims of your presentation will vary according to the purpose of the presentation, the topic, and the audience.

Aims in relation to health care include:

- prevention
- rehabilitation
- education
- health promotion.

Other general aims include:

- dissemination of information
- stimulation of debate
- persuasion
- decision making
- negotiating a contract.

Increasing numbers of health care courses now include specific training on communication skills. As a student you may have been required to make a presentation as part of your assessment. As you progress from student to clinician, and perhaps into management, your work may involve you in leading workshops or giving presentations to colleagues. Whether you remain in clinical work or move into management you will have to deal with a variety of audiences. Each one will require a different presentation format and style of delivery. Some examples of presentations given by health professionals are:

- *Support group* for parents of children with Down's Syndrome
- *Presenting a research paper* at a conference
- *Running a workshop* on first aid

- ○ *Lecturing* undergraduate students
- ○ *Presenting information* on service delivery to the purchasing authority
- ○ Participating in a research *seminar*
- ○ *Training* careworkers in lifting and handling elderly clients.

What sort of presentations are you involved in delivering?

The main part of this section looks at presentation skills in general. It includes the following topics:

Preparation

Essential things you need to know before you begin. Making a draft of your presentation. Getting the timing right on the day. Tips on making your presentation more interesting.

Effective use of the voice

Review of the anatomy and physiology of voice production. Eliminating the 'nervous' voice. Using your voice as a presentation tool. Tips on taking care of your voice. Practical exercises for the voice.

Delivering content

Getting the message across. Dealing with questions. Supporting the spoken word.

Using non-verbal communication

Using eye-contact, gesture and body language to help communicate your message. Annoying habits and what to do about them.

Establishing rapport with the audience

Tips on getting the audience on your side. Learning to 'read' the audience. Making an exit.

Effective use of audio-visual aids

Types of audio-visual aids available to the presenter. Choosing the appropriate aids. Hints on using and preparing audio-visual materials. Checklist of audio-visual aids.

The final part of this section looks at different kinds of presentations. Use these sections for specific advice regarding presentations in these contexts:

Client/carer workshops

Running a workshop. Ideas for activities including behavioural rehearsal and role play. Giving participants feedback. Using demonstration to teach a skill.

Presentations to other professionals

Why these presentations are challenging. Avoiding the pitfalls. Calming the nerves. Positive aspects.

Lectures

Structuring your lecture. Teaching and learning strategies. Activities to promote student participation. Student evaluation forms for lectures.

Selling your Service

The art of persuasion. Tips on presentation. Working as a team.

Presenting your Research

Making your presentation memorable. How to present your numerical information effectively. Checklist for presenting research.

16

Preparation

A presentation is like an iceberg. The delivery is only the tip of this iceberg. Nine-tenths is preparation. You would not dream of building a house without foundations. In the same way it is dangerous to rely on your ability to ad-lib on the day. A solid base of preparation lies beneath every successful performance. The well-prepared presentation demonstrates that you value the audience, and respect their time and attention. It will also give you a sense of security.

Before embarking on the main stages of preparation, you need to find out the:

- Who?
- What?
- Where?
- and When?

Who is your audience?

Ask the organisers for approximate numbers, and a list of names and occupations if this is available. You need to establish information about their specific needs and requirements. This can be determined to some extent by the type of presentation. For example, your expectations about theoretical knowledge would differ considerably between post-graduate and under-graduate students. The reason for attendance will give you some idea about their motivation. Is attendance a compulsory component of their course or an extra-curricular activity? Some course organisers ask participants to complete a questionnaire about their expectations of the course. You might consider asking participants to complete a form in advance.

Aim to find out the following information:

- Knowledge and experience of your topic area and other related fields

- ○ Attitudes (this includes attitudes to health care, health professionals, as well as attitudes to learning and attending courses)
- ○ Motivation for attending (Is their attendance voluntary or were they directed to attend the course?)
- ○ Level of interest (What do they hope to gain from the presentation? How relevant is the topic to their work? Is this part of an accredited course ending in a qualification?)

This information will help you to decide what content is relevant for this audience and the best way to convey it.

What is the purpose and nature of the presentation?

Unfortunately, asking the organiser to specify the purpose of the talk often elicits vague comments like, 'the students need some background to their theory lectures' or 'we would like to hear about some research.' It is often more enlightening to ask why you in particular were approached as a speaker. Try to establish which of the areas in your topic are core. Find out how much detail the organisers are expecting.

At this stage it is important to say whether you feel it is appropriate for you to do the presentation. Another colleague may have more experience in this area. If this is the case then pass the request on to them.

Find out what format the presentation will take. Is it expected to be formal or informal? This will be determined to some extent by the venue and the purpose of the presentation. The organisers may also have ideas about style of delivery. They might want to encourage interaction with the audience, or keep presentations brief with questions reserved to the end of a morning or afternoon. This will affect content and delivery. For example a formal presentation may have a chairperson to field questions. An informal work-shop requires practical activities.

Where is the venue?

Find out the location of your venue. Never assume that the name of the building indicates its precise whereabouts. Charing Cross Hospital is in Hammersmith not Charing Cross Road. Do not leave it to the last minute to confirm these travel details!

Check your accommodation. There is no point in planning small group activities if you have to work in a tiered lecture theatre. You will also need to know something about the acoustics, particularly if you are talking to a large audience. Find out the lay-out of the room, type of seating and what audio-visual aids are available. Is amplification required? Which audio-visual aids are appropriate? You need to know all of these things before you can start any planning.

When is the presentation?

Find out the date and time for your presentation and agree on the length of your session. Your presentation may be one of several, either during a day or over a period of days. Try to avoid difficult slots like the session after lunch or last thing on a Friday afternoon when people are tired or want to go home. Find out what talks come before and after your slot. This will help you avoid repetition and link your content to other presentations.

Once you have this information you can draw up a schedule for your preparation. List all your jobs with the dates for completion. (See *Checklist for Preparation*.) Some examples of tasks are:

- reading up on your subject area
- writing out notes
- drafting your presentation
- preparing audio-visual aids
- preparing and photocopying handouts
- rehearsing your presentation.

Aim to complete your preparation at least a week before your presentation. Remember to allow time to photocopy materials. Agree a schedule with other staff who are helping with the preparation. Put in a time margin for checking and correcting errors. The final item on your time plan is your dress rehearsal.

Deciding on your content

The content of your presentation may be novel information, as with research; or established facts and theories. Some information may be specific, and therefore very easy to define in a plan. Other topics may be less predictable, particularly if the audience have a role in shaping the agenda. Whatever your presentation, the first step is to identify the core content, and to draw up a draft plan. How you prepare this draft is very much a question of individual style. However, there are some general principles you can apply.

Start by making sure you are clear about the purpose of your presentation. Scriptwriters are advised to condense their story ideas into one sentence (Hauge 1989). This is a useful technique for presentations. Write out the purpose of your talk in one sentence. You may need several attempts before you are satisfied that you have a succinct and clear statement. Use a series of questions to refine your objective. For example, take an original idea of a talk about 'stopping smoking' Who is it targeting? Why should people want to stop smoking? How can they be persuaded? Your statement may end up as – 'To convince adolescents of the benefits of not smoking and to inform them of the options available for breaking the habit'.

Your objective forms the starting point for drafting the content of your talk. The aims of a draft are to ensure that you have:

(1) All the information required to meet your objective

(2) A plan for conveying this information in a logical and interesting fashion.

Here are some suggestions of ways in which you can develop ideas for your presentation.

Brainstorm the topic. Write down all your thoughts related to your objective on a large piece of paper (poster size). Use words and short phrases, as speed is the essence. Instead of writing lines across the page or listing items down the page, leave spaces around each point so you can group related items together. In this way you are starting to sort and categorise your thoughts as you go along.

Once you have exhausted your ideas you can start to highlight key concepts by circling or underlining them. Write these on a separate piece of paper, spacing them well apart. Either circle or draw a box around each one. Ideas from your first brainstorm can be listed under these key concepts using a spider's web design, (see Figure 4.1).

Once you have collated all the points, you can think about ordering them according to whether they are a primary or a secondary point. Eventually you will end up with your original brainstorm divided into categories. For example (see Figure 4.2)

An alternative approach is to make a list of the key concepts you want to cover.

For example

Key concepts:

◊ Effects of Smoking

◊ Benefits of Stopping Smoking

◊ Ways of Breaking the Addiction

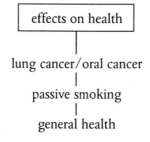

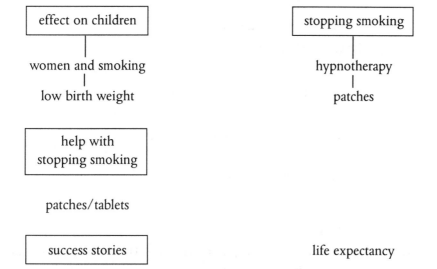

Figure 4.1 An example of brainstorm on the topic of 'stopping smoking'

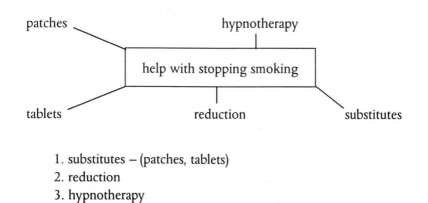

1. substitutes – (patches, tablets)
2. reduction
3. hypnotherapy

Figure 4.2 Prioritising points from a spider's web

Next, list ideas or topics under the appropriate heading. Be careful not to swamp the main points with too much detail. Eventually you will have the skeleton of your talk.

For example

- ◊ Effects of Smoking
    - ◦ lung and heart disease; link with other illnesses
    - ◦ personal hygiene (bad breath, nicotine stains)
    - ◦ social acceptance
    - ◦ effects on the health of others.
- ◊ Benefits of Stopping
    - ◦ save money
    - ◦ healthier
    - ◦ social acceptance.
- ◊ Ways of Breaking the Addiction
    - ◦ patches
    - ◦ pills
    - ◦ hypnotherapy
    - ◦ support groups.

You now have the main points of your presentation. Use these to guide your background reading and note-taking.

Structuring your presentation

The next stage is to put your material into a logical sequence.

Wilder (1990) suggests the following structure:

- ◦ An introduction
- ◦ An opening statement that sets the tone of the presentation
- ◦ An outline of the main points
- ◦ An in-depth exploration of the main points
- ◦ A summary (and recommendations).

This standard format will vary according to the purpose or aims of your presentation. Think about what you want to achieve with your audience. Look at the following examples:

Aim	Result

To *teach* a skill   Audience to *learn* a skill

How will your presentation help these people to learn a skill? You might employ demonstrations, explanations and practical experience.

To *sell* a service   Audience to *buy* a service

How will your presentation persuade the audience to buy your service? You might discuss the benefits of your service to the audience, and prepare arguments to counter objections.

To *share* information   Audience to *understand* and
                                                  remember information

The emphasis will be on presenting the information clearly and succinctly in a way that will be memorable for the audience. This type of presentation is appropriate for sharing research findings or presenting annual reports.

To *teach* theory   Audience to *increase knowledge*
                                                  and *comprehension*

Teaching involves presenting ideas, facts and arguments.

To *entertain*   Audience to *enjoy*

You might think this is an aim for every presentation, but there are occasions where a presentation is purely for entertainment. This may be an introduction to a fund raising event or an after dinner speech. You are more likely to use humour, anecdotes and interesting stories.

When you start to apply your format, you may find you have additional points to add. At this stage you can also check your draft for repetition, controversial points or irrelevant items.

Determining your delivery

Once you know what you are going to say, you can start thinking about the best way of getting your message across. Again, how you deliver your presentation will depend on your aims. A lecture will require explanations, a workshop will involve practical demonstrations and presenting a research paper requires reporting skills. Look at the chapter on *Presentation Skills in Context* for specific guidance for your presentation.

Attention curve

The attention and concentration of your audience will not remain at the same level throughout your presentation. Attention tends to decrease after the first ten minutes (Bligh 1983). It continues to fall until it reaches the lowest point half-an-hour into your presentation. To counteract this effect you need to use attention gaining devices such as showing an overhead, varying your presentation style, or answering some questions (Gibbs 1992). If the audience know your finishing time their attention will start to rise again five minutes before this. This makes it a good time to summarise your main points.

Using audio-visual aids

Find out what audio-visual aids are available at the venue before you start your planning. The organisers may be able to get equipment especially for your presentation, but do not rely on this until it has been confirmed.

You may be wondering why you need to bother with audio-visual aids. A quick look at their contribution to presentations will persuade you that the benefits justify the time and effort involved in their preparation.

A visual image can instantly:

○ Express a message – 'children smoking pretend cigarettes'

○ Illustrate an idea – 'plan of a new clinic'

○ Explain a concept – 'oxygenation of the blood'

The information contained in one simple visual may take a page of text to explain. Research has also shown that visual aids help increase the audience's understanding, interest and attention span, as well as aiding memory and providing structure both for the audience and the presenter.

Similarly, it may be difficult to describe in words a predominantely auditory event, such as the effects of ageing on the voice or the characteristics of speech in schizophrenia. Use sound without picture to create a dramatic effect. This is exactly what a television documentary did. They recorded the removal of bandages from a severely burned boy. There was sound but the screen was blank. The audience were focused totally on the cries of pain and suffering.

Many audio visual aids combine auditory and visual images. Video is commonly available and with the advent of multi-media it is possible to combine text, video and audio on the computer screen. We know that people remember only 10 per cent of what they read and 20 per cent of what they hear. They are likely to remember 30 per cent from visual images, which is increased to 50 per cent when this is combined with listening. During conversation 7 per cent is communicated verbally while 38 per cent is how we say it and 55 per cent is what we see (Bunch 1995). If you want to get your message across, *say* it and *show* it.

There are also benefits for the presenter who uses aids. Visuals shift the attention of the audience away from the speaker, who then has some thinking time or a moment to relax. They can act as an aide-memoire and provide a structure for the talk. Presenters who use visual aids are perceived as more competent and professional (The 3M Meeting Management Team 1994).

Look through your draft and identify where you may be able to use audio-visual aids. Use them at points when the audience's concentration is low; this is usually during the middle and second half of a talk. It also helps maintain interest if you vary the types of audio-visual aid you use during the presentation. Intersperse your overheads with a video clip and a practical demonstration using an anatomical model.

Remember the visual is there to reinforce the verbal message, not to provide a written duplicate of your presentation. Always ask yourself – is this slide or acetate necessary? It must add information, help explain a point, or illustrate the message you are trying to convey through speech. Never use an acetate or slide that regurgitates what you have said in written form.

Timing

Once you have your overall structure you can start to think about timing. This is often a problem for even experienced speakers. Although people worry about not having enough to say, in reality speakers often over run. Bad time-keeping upsets the whole programme of a course or conference, and results in other speakers having to curtail their presentations. This does not win points in the popularity stakes with either presenters or the audience.

Build a time-table into your presentation during the preparation stage. Estimate how long it will take to cover each section. Remember to include timings for using audio-visual aids, answering questions and setting up demonstrations.

If your presentation proceeds at a quicker pace than expected, it is useful to have a few extra items up your sleeve. These can be slotted in at the appropriate place. Choose information that is not central to your presentation, but would be of interest if time allows. If your presentation is taking longer than planned, it is useful to have identified in advance sections that can be omitted without destroying the structure of your presentation or distorting your message. In the normal course of events, these sections would be included in the presentation. The remaining sections form the core or absolute minimum for your presentation.

Write out your plan as if all the sections are to be included. Mark which sections may be omitted or added using a code. For example:

Ø Omit if short of time

→ Additional section if not enough material

These classifications are for your private use only. Do not tell the audience about items you would like to include if you had the time. What the ear does not hear the heart will not miss!

Finishing the presentation

The ending of your presentation is just as important as the beginning. Time your presentation carefully so that you do not just tail off at the end. The way that you finish will relate directly to your opening statements and your aims. It will always have a summary of the main points and usually some recommendations. Do not include new information in your summing up.

Aides-memoire

Most good speakers use some form of aide-memoire during their talk. An aide-memoire provides a reminder of the general structure of the talk. Some people prefer to write key points on small cards that are held in the palm of the hand. Other people prefer to write out more detailed information on sheets of paper. What ever method you choose, number the pages or cards. This will help you sort them quickly if they are dropped. You may want to secure cards and paper with treasury tags.

Hints on preparing aides-memoire:

- Notes must be readable. Write clearly so that words can be read at a distance, for example if your notes are laid out on a table.

- Write down the time that each section will take and include a running total. For example, after two 15 minute sections your running total will be half an hour. This can be represented in real time. If your start time was two o'clock your running time would be two-thirty. This way you can instantly check if you are ahead or behind in your overall timing.

- Add notation to indicate which sections can be omitted. See 'timing' above.

- Use icons to indicate where you plan to use audio-visual aids. You can also show where you want to use examples, demonstrations and anecdotes.

○ Make the structure of your talk clear by highlighting headings and separating sections. Leave space to add in amendments at the last minute.

Final dress rehearsal

Try to carry out your dress rehearsal in the same location as your presentation. If this is not possible, then simulate the surroundings by replicating the lay-out of chairs and using the same room size. Run through the presentation using your planned audio-visual aids. Avoid stopping as you need to get a feel for how the presentation comes across as a whole.

This type of practice is crucial if your presentation is part of a team. All team members need to rehearse together. There may still be final adjustments to make at this stage, particularly with timing. Team members can make notes about each other's performance.

If you are presenting alone, ask a friend or colleague to be a member of your audience. You need feedback, particularly on timing, clarity, repetition and overall interest. Somebody who is familiar with the reactions of your audience will be able to detect any controversial statements.

CHECKLIST FOR PREPARATION

Type of Accommodation:

> **Title of Presentation:**
>
> **Date:**   **Time:**   **Length:**
> **Name/Address of Venue**

Travel arrangements confirmed

Type of presentation

□ Lecture   □ Workshop   □ Seminar   □ Conference
□ Presentation

Planning Schedule

	Date	Subgoals

Goal _____

                                   1 ....

                                   2 ....

                                   3 ....

Goal _____

                                   1 ....

                                   2 ....

                                   3 ....

Goal _____

                                   1 ....

                                   2 ....

                                   3 ....

Goal _____

                                   1 ....

                                   2 ....

                                   3 ....

Name of Organiser:

Contact address and tel. No.:

Date for completion

Action Points

(1) Rehearse your presentation, including the use of audio-visual aids. Check your timing.

(2) Ask a friend or family member to give you some constructive advice. Were your ideas presented well? Did they enjoy the anecdotes? How clear were the graphics?

Different listeners provide alternative perspectives. A naive listener, who has no specialist knowledge of the area, will appreciate clear explanations but is less likely to spot errors or inaccuracies. An experienced listener will know the subject very well but they may fail to recognise when an explanation is inadequate.

Remember to ask for positive feedback and suggestions for solutions.

(3) Video or audio record yourself to see and hear yourself as the audience do. It is always a shock to hear your voice on tape or see yourself on camera for the first time. Remember your nose is not really that crooked, your accent is not that strong or your tummy that large in real life! Remember the camera tends to add a couple of pounds.

(4) Once you have given a presentation you will be much better prepared for next time. You will have more idea about what works and what is less successful. Make a note of items that worked well, and any changes needed for future presentations.

Summary Points

- A presentation is like an iceberg with nine-tenths hidden from the audience. This is the preparation stage, which is essential for a successful presentation.

- Get to know your audience. Find out about their knowledge, experience, skills, attitudes and needs.

- Establish the purpose and the nature of your presentation.

- Check on accommodation and time-table details. Find out who is before and after you in the programme.

- Plan your preparation well in advance. Use a schedule that lists all the jobs with the completion dates.

- Structure the content of your presentation according to your aims and the nature of the presentation.

- Decide how you will deliver the content. This will vary according to your aims.

- Plan your presentation to follow the attention curve of the audience. Attention is greatest at the start and the end of a presentation.

- Use a variety of audio-visual aids to add interest and help you to get your message across.

- Plan the timing of your presentation. Identify sections that can be added or omitted as necessary. Do not forget your ending. Summarise your main points and include any recommendations.

- Prepare aides-memoire on cards or paper. Use notation to indicate where you want to use audio-visual aids, examples and so on.

- Your last preparation task is the dress rehearsal. Ask a friend or another presenter to comment on the performance. Amend your script as necessary.

17

Effective Use of Voice

In a presentation the main mode of communication is oral. The message is delivered through the spoken word, supported by visual aids such as overheads or video. When we read a book the message is conveyed through the written word, with diagrams and drawings used to illustrate the text. The difference with a presentation is that the effective speaker can use the voice as another presentation tool. Variations in tone, pitch or volume emphasise key points. A well-placed pause builds anticipation. An expressive voice captures the attention of the listeners.

Making a presentation is often equated with giving a performance. *How* you say your message becomes just as important as *what* you are saying. The description 'performance' may set your nerves jangling, especially if you are inexperienced at public speaking. The voice is affected by how you are feeling (Hirano 1981). Nerves may manifest themselves in a wavery pitch, volume being too quiet or too loud, or the voice suddenly deserting the speaker altogether. Using the voice effectively is a common concern for many novice presenters.

Effective use of the voice involves:

(1) Understanding how voice is produced

(2) Developing your voice as a performance tool

(3) Learning how to care for your voice.

(1) Understanding how voice is produced

Introduction

Voice is the result of complex physiological processes that depend on the appropriate anatomical structures functioning efficiently. Any abnormalities of these structures or deficiencies in functional ability will affect the development and quality of speech. For the listener, voice is an auditory event whose characteristics are described in acoustic terms, so that we think about the pitch, tone and volume of the speaker's voice. Audition also enables us to monitor our voice. Without auditory feedback we would find it difficult to maintain our voices at appropriate levels and over time quality and tone would deteriorate. Voice is a sound that we make using structures in the larynx. To understand how we produce it, we first need to have some understanding of how a sound is made.

How a sound is made?

Borden and Harris (1980, p.33) define a sound as an 'audible disturbance of a medium produced by a source'. What exactly does this mean?

We can use the guitar as an example of how a sound occurs. When the strings of the guitar are plucked, they are set into motion or, in other words, they vibrate. However, this is not the sound that we hear when a guitar is played. The vibrating string makes very little sound itself. Instead the vibrations from the string set the air contained within the hollow body of the guitar into motion. The wooden body of the guitar acts like a resonator, making the sounds richer and louder.

The movement of air molecules inside the guitar causes the molecules in the surrounding air to be displaced. These disturbances form a wave or set of movements that spread out from the guitar. When these movements or sound waves reach the human ear they cause the ear drum to vibrate. These vibrations pass through the ear to the organ of hearing, which lies within the inner ear. The sound is analysed into its component frequencies and transmitted to the cortex through the auditory nerve.

So before we can make a sound we need a source, a form of propulsion to set the source into motion, and a medium for transmitting these vibrations. In the above example the source of the sound is the guitar string, and the medium is the surrounding air. The vibrations of the source, brought about by plucking the guitar string, cause a disturbance in the surrounding medium. Air is not the only medium for transmitting sound. Any gas, liquid or solid object can act as a medium. We can hear sound underwater and metal pipes transmit tapping.

Some sound waves are not audible to the human ear, for example the high pitched dog whistle. This is because they fail to cause a vibration in the human auditory system. For sound to be audible, the vibrations need to be capable of setting off complementary vibrations in the receiving auditory system (Borden and Harris 1980).

This explains how a sound is made, but how is voice produced? The following sections review the anatomy and physiology of the structures involved in phonation, and examine the production of voice in more detail.

Review of anatomy and physiology

The structures involved in phonation are the lungs, the vocal folds and the vocal tract.

The lungs

The two lungs lie within the thoracic cavity. This cavity is formed by the rib cage, by the sternum at the front and by the vertebral column at the back. A large dome shaped muscle sheet, called the diaphragm, separates the thoracic cavity from the abdominal cavity. The lungs are conical in shape with their base resting on the diaphragm. They consist of porous, spongy and very elastic air cells (Kaplan 1960). The nature of the tissue means that the contour of the lungs is moulded by the thoracic cavity, although the basic conical shape is maintained. In addition, a membranous connection between the

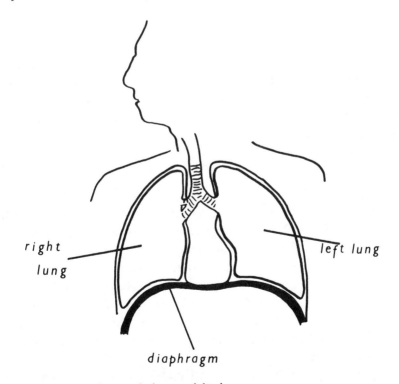

Figure 4.3 Diagram showing the lungs and diaphragm

lungs and the thoracic cavity allows movement of it as a whole (Martin 1987). The lungs have two functions, one is respiration and the other is phonation.

The vocal folds

The airstream for respiration enters and exits from the lungs through the larynx, within which lie the vocal folds. There are two sets of folds: the true vocal folds and the false vocal folds. In normal speech only the true folds are involved in phonation (Bunch 1982). They are positioned behind the thyroid cartilage, which can be felt in the throat as the Adam's apple or voice box.

The folds are membranous protuberances that stretch across the larynx and are capable of forming a closure similar in operation to a valve. However, the folds are not simply sphincteric in function (Borden and Harris 1980). They have several sets of muscles that allow them to alter their shape and tension. The folds can be elongated, made shorter or thickened. Each fold is covered with mucous membrane, which is loose and movable like the skin on the back of the hand (Baken 1991).

The vocal tract

The vocal tract is the term for all the air passages above the vocal folds, including the pharyngeal cavity, the oral cavity and the nasal cavity. Parts of the tract are muscular and capable of very fast movements (Bunch 1982). It is possible to change the shape, size and tension of the vocal tract. It can be made longer or shorter, and its width altered. These cavities function as resonators.

Production of voice

Breath support for speech

The vocal folds are the sound source of voice. In order to produce voice we need a form of propulsion or energy to set this sound source into motion. This is supplied by the airstream from the lungs.

During normal respiration air is inspired when the pressure within the thoracic cavity, and concomitantly within the lungs, is lowered. This occurs when the cavity is enlarged by the contraction of the diaphragm and the elevation of the ribs. Air is sucked into the lungs, which expand due to the elastic nature of their cells, until the internal pressure is equalised with the atmospheric pressure.

Expiration is largely passive, with the main force provided by the recoiling of the now inflated lungs, and the rib cage. This occurs when the

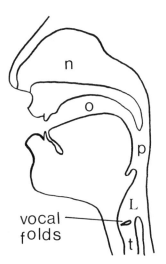

key:

N – nasal cavity

O – oral cavity

p – pharynx

L – larynx

t – trachea

Figure 4.4 The vocal tract

diaphragm and other inspiratory muscles relax, decreasing the volume of the thoracic cavity and the lungs. This causes the pressure to increase and air is exhaled.

This process of inspiration and expiration alters during speech. Unlike respiration, which is under automatic control, breathing for speech involves voluntary control. In contrast to normal breathing the inspiration phase is quicker, with a longer expiratory phase. A greater volume of air is required and this is achieved by the use of additional muscles to elevate the sternum and ribs. In expiration extra muscle control is used to sustain voicing. Muscles, usually used for inspiration, help control airflow out of the lungs. There is also greater airflow through the mouth during expiration, rather than the nose, which is usual during normal respiration.

Voicing

At rest the vocal folds are apart and the v-shaped space between them is called the glottis (Perkins and Kent 1986). The folds do not vibrate in this open position. Just before phonation the vocal folds are adducted or brought together, causing pressure to build up in the airstream from the lungs. Eventually this pressure forces the folds apart in an upward and outward movement from bottom to top. As the airstream passes through the fortis the pressure starts to drop and the folds begin to close, this time from top to bottom. The whole process is assisted by the elastic nature of the folds. These intermittent closures chop the airstream into short bursts (Baken 1991). As the air passes across the surface of the vocal folds they are caused to vibrate, with the loosely attached mucus membrane tending to undulate in waves (Perkins and Kent 1986). The result of this vibration is phonation.

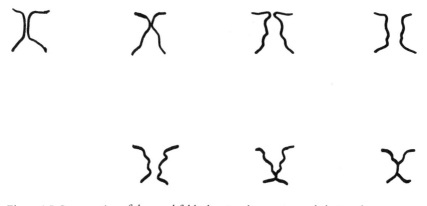

Figure 4.5 Cross-section of the vocal folds showing the opening and closing phases.

The sound produced by the vibration of the vocal folds is not the actual sound we hear and recognise as voice. The laryngeal mechanism supplies only the raw material. This basic sound is amplified by the resonating cavities of the vocal tract. These resonators are also responsible for giving a speaker's voice its characteristic tone and richness.

The laryngeal mechanism is involved in determining pitch and intonation. The number of glottal openings per second is known as the fundamental frequency (Denes and Pinson 1973). Although the voice consists of many frequencies, it is the fundamental frequency, or lowest frequency, of the voice that the listener perceives as the speaker's pitch. Male and female voices differ in pitch, partly because of the difference in size of the larynx. The fundamental frequency for a male speaker is usually between 100 and 160 Hz, and for a female between 220 and 290 Hz (Fawcus 1986). Changes in vocal fold tension, mass and elasticity also affect frequency. For example, the frequency of vibration is increased when the folds become tense. During speech the fundamental frequency is continually changing to produce the pitch movements associated with various intonation patterns.

Articulation

It is not possible to consider phonation without examining the role of articulation. The articulators are the lips, the tongue, the soft palate and the teeth. They are involved in altering the resonance of the vocal tract by altering its length, size and shape. For example when the lips are protruded for the sound 'oo', the tract is made longer.

In English we can divide speech sounds into two groups. *Voiced* sounds occur when the vocal folds are vibrating (the process described above). *Voiceless* sounds are produced when the vocal folds are open. The air passes through the fortis without restriction; the source of the sound is higher up in the vocal tract.

You can feel the vibrations of a voiced sound by placing your fingertips on either side of your Adam's apple and saying 'ah'. Compare this sensation with the one you get when you produce a long 's'. You will find that 'ah' is a voiced sound, as are all vowels. The consonant 's' is a voiceless sound. The sound source is in the vocal tract, above the level of the vocal folds. Consonants can be voiced or voiceless. Try pairs of sounds like 'p' and 'b', 't' and 'd' or 'k' and 'g'. Be careful you only say the sound and do not add a vowel as in 'per' or 'pea'. Otherwise the voicing of the vowel will mask any voiceless sounds.

Movements of the articulators produce speech sounds by controlling the airstream by either constricting or blocking the vocal tract. You will find that some sounds are produced by a movement of the articulators that form a closure in the vocal tract. The sound 'p' is formed by the bringing together of the lips. Air pressure builds up behind the closure and is released in an explosive burst. These sounds are known, not surprisingly, as plosives. They include p, b, t, d, k, and g.

Another group of sounds is known as fricatives. They are produced when the airstream is forced through a narrow constriction in the vocal tract. The sound 's' is a fricative. It can be made by placing the tip of the tongue behind the top teeth. A small gap is left between the tongue and the alveolar ridge (the ridge behind your top teeth). Air is forced in a continuous flow through the gap creating friction. The result is the characteristic 's' sound. Fricatives can be voiced or voiceless. Try the sound 'z'. You will find there are two sources of sound. One at the vocal folds and the other in the oral cavity. Fricatives include the sounds f, v, and sh. As with voiced sounds, a voiceless sound is resonated in the cavities of the vocal tract.

Summary Points

○ The airstream from the lungs supplies the propulsion or energy which sets the vocal folds into vibration. The basic sound produced by these vibrations is amplified by the resonating cavities of the vocal tract. These resonators also add tone and warmth to the voice.

○ Speech sounds are formed by modifications to the airstream caused by movements of the articulators. Sounds can be voiced (vocal folds are vibrating) or voiceless (vocal folds are open).

(2) Developing your voice as a performance tool

Your voice is a significant channel for communicating your message. The audience are there to listen to you, the speaker. Although your presentation may include visual aids and handouts, the audience do not want to read a book or watch a film. These are activities they can do by themselves. You are there to give your views, share your knowledge, explain ideas and help the audience understand the issues. The audience are interested in you as a speaker.

When you have a conversation you usually take turns at speaking. But when you are giving a presentation you have the responsibility for the majority of the speaking time. For the audience there is more emphasis on listening, and so greater attention is paid to the voice characteristics of the speaker. Making the voice interesting and pleasant is therefore essential.

Using your voice effectively is about control and manipulation. First there are some basic techniques that you need to master before you can start to use your voice creatively. You need to be able to make yourself heard by everybody in the audience, and to deliver your speech with clarity, at an appropriate pace. The following sections look at exactly what you need to do.

Relaxation

Tension is a natural characteristic of the body. Without it we would collapse in a heap and be unable to move. We need a certain amount of muscle tone to maintain our posture, and movements of our body rely on the contraction and relaxation of our muscles. However, excessive tension is tiring and affects the efficient functioning of the body. Underlying all voice techniques is the ability to relax. Relaxation focuses on reducing the excess tension and thereby improving vocal quality. Use the practical exercises at the end of this section to help you relax. These include suggestions on making a relaxation tape.

Audibility

The fundamental requirement of the speaker is to be audible. It is also true that an inappropriately loud voice can be grating for an audience, almost like a physical assault. But for most people the problem is that their voice is too quiet or their speech is mumbled. Audibility is not necessarily about volume although an adequate level needs to be achieved. This level will vary according to the size of the audience and the acoustics of the room. Posture, breathing, resonance, projection, and clarity of articulation greatly assist the speaker's efforts to improve audibility. Let's look at each of these areas and how they contribute to the overall delivery by the speaker.

Posture and breathing patterns

As we have seen above, phonation relies on the pulmonic egressive airstream, which means basically that sounds of the English language are made using air that is breathed out of the lungs. If this air runs out then the speaker has no means to continue phonation. You can try this for yourself by counting (one, two, three...) on one breath until you run out of air. You will notice the voice gets weaker and quieter, and eventually stops when all the air has been used.

Normally the speaker will make sure that enough air is taken in to produce speech. However, problems occur when the speaker is anxious or nervous. Breathing can become shallow with the intake of air insufficient, resulting in a loss of volume and deterioration of quality. Some speakers may even 'forget' to breathe out, holding their breath while speaking, as if they were about to plunge into a pool. This has the same undesirable effect on the voice as not having enough air.

To establish good breathing habits you need to start with a posture that encourages maximum use of lung capacity. A position that restricts movement of the thorax, and particularly the diaphragm, is to be avoided. Standing or sitting with your shoulders hunched and your back bowed will result in tension in the neck area. Try this position, and then compare this with one where the back is straight and the head balanced in the mid line. You will find your shoulders are relaxed and the chest area is spread rather than squashed. There are practical exercises at the end of this section to help you develop the best posture.

Once you have established a good posture you can work on your breathing. Watch yourself in a mirror. Which parts of your upper body move as you breathe in and out? If you can see the upper chest moving and the shoulders rising excessively with each breath, you are probably using a type of breathing known as clavicular. It is often seen in people who are exerting themselves, or in people who are fearful or nervous. For speech, it is a less efficient method of breathing.

Good breathing patterns work with the natural forces of respiration. Avoid taking deep breaths or gulping in air. Breathing needs to expand the lower part of the lungs. Concentrate your efforts here. Remember the diaphragm also plays an essential role in breathing. Thoracic and lung volume are increased and decreased by its contraction and relaxation. These movements are helped by a relaxed and balanced posture. A full description of diaphragmatic breathing is provided in the practical section at the end.

Projection

How can you make sure that your voice is heard at the back of a large auditorium? Although adequate volume is essential as a starting point, projecting your voice is not just about speaking loudly. Start by thinking about who you are addressing in the audience. Are you talking to the people in the front row? The middle row? Or the back row? We naturally adjust our voices to suit the distance. Try this practical exercise to develop a feel for these changes. Speak to an imaginary person. Compare your voice when this person is next to you, at the other side of the room and then outside the room. Posture will also affect your ability to project your voice. The position of your upper body is crucial. Listen to the difference in the sound of your voice when you count to twenty with your chin tucked on your chest, and when you count with your head up. Aim to keep your head centred in the middle (looking straight ahead) and the jaw area relaxed. Be careful that your head does not tilt backwards or your chin lift up. This is counter productive as it creates tension in the neck area, and adversely affects voice quality. If this habit continues over time it can also lead to voice problems.

Look around at your audience, rather than speaking down to the floor or at your notes. This encourages an upright position of the head, which will help your voice to carry. Your audience should be able to look into your eyes, not be staring at the parting in your hair!

Another technique in voice projection is maximising the resonance of the voice. Within the vocal tract there are several cavities that function as resonators. As a speaker it is easier to think of these areas as the mouth, nose and throat. These resonators naturally amplify the sound produced by our vocal folds. A voice with a full resonance will carry further than one that is thin and lacking in resonance. You can help your resonating cavities to work efficiently by relaxing the head and neck area. There are also specific practical exercises for improving resonance at the end of this section.

There is a tendency for speakers to slow down their speech when they concentrate on projecting their voices. Voices may also become flat and lack expressiveness. Practise projecting your voice whilst still maintaining the normal pace and rhythm of your speech.

Clarity

Slurred words or mumbled phrases are difficult to understand in any situation. When speaking to a large number of people, rather than a group of friends, more precise articulation is required. This does not mean exaggerating each word. If you do, you will sound odd, and alter the natural rhythm of speech. The aim is to increase accuracy.

Be careful that your efforts do not create too much tension in the face and jaw. Instead aim to increase the strength of your articulation. Compare the difference in tension between a gentle pout and pursing the lips, or a half-hearted smile and a grimace with lips spread. Try making some 'b b b' sounds, bringing the lips together with exaggerated force. Feel the tension in your throat and lips this has created. Now make the same sounds by bringing the lips together lightly, so that articulation is precise but the mouth and throat are relaxed. See the section on 'articulation exercises' for more ideas to improve the clarity of your speech.

One final point on articulation. It is often confused with elocution, with people encouraged to speak in 'proper English'. Never feel obliged to adopt any accent that is not your own. This is unnecessary, and is likely to interrupt your flow of ideas, as you concentrate on your pronunciation of each word. Always be yourself.

Pace

The clarity of your speech is closely linked to the rate at which you speak. If the pace is too fast it will be difficult to maintain precise articulation. The audience may also have difficulty in keeping up with you, especially if your material is unfamiliar or complex. Sometimes it is the converse problem of a speaker being too slow in their delivery. Spoken language follows a natural rhythm, which can become distorted if the pace slows down too much.

Try reading aloud a passage from the newspaper in a number of different speaker styles. For example:

- The 'Hey man. I'm so laid back' speaker
- The 'deliberate (definitely no mistakes here)' speaker
- The 'If I rush the next bit they might not notice my mistakes' speaker
- The 'I want to get this over with as soon as possible' speaker.

Compare the different rates of speaking. Now read aloud the passage using an appropriate pace. The chapter on *Delivering Content* has more advice on pacing your delivery.

Using your voice as a performance tool

Like your audio-visual aids and your handouts, your voice is another tool in your presentation kit. Here are some ideas of different ways the voice can be used in a presentation:

- Raise your voice or change the pitch to gain the audience's attention. You can revert to normal once they are attending.
- Use an expressive voice that varies rhythm and pitch to add interest (Rosenshine 1971). The voice often becomes more lively when the speaker tells an anecdote or gives an opinion. Intersperse factual material with plenty of examples, analogies, and stories.
- Learn to use the tone of your voice to tell the audience how you feel about a subject or to indicate your attitude to an issue.
- Emphasise important words or phrases by varying volume, slowing down or changing the intonation patterns.
- Experiment with using different intonation patterns in your explanations.

Summary Points

- The voice is the main medium of communication in a presentation. The audience have to spend a greater amount of time listening, so speaker characteristics take on more significance.

- Relaxation is the key to all voice techniques. Excessive tension will affect vocal quality.

- All speakers need to be audible. But audibility is not just about increasing volume. Breathing, posture, resonance, projection and clarity are all important in helping you to be heard.

- The correct posture will help you establish good breathing patterns. The body needs to be balanced and symmetrical with the head in the midline and the back straight.

- Good breathing patterns work with the natural forces of respiration. Concentrate on expanding the lower part of the chest.

- Think about where you want to project your voice. Speak to the back row. Your voice will naturally adjust to the distance.

- Your voice will carry better if your head is up and you are looking at the audience. Avoid lifting the chin as this creates strain in the neck area.

- Remember to keep some variation in your pitch when you are projecting your voice.

- Improve the precision of your articulation without increasing the tension or exaggerating your speech.

- Maintain an appropriate pace of speech. If it is too fast the audience will have difficulty in understanding. If it is too slow the natural rhythm is altered.

- Use your voice as another performance tool. It can add interest, maintain concentration and provide emphasis.

(3) Learning how to care for your voice

Your voice is an instrument and like any other instrument it needs care and attention. In everyday life the voice may be affected by a number of different circumstances. Everybody will have experienced the 'croaky voice' following an evening of over-indulgence in alcohol and smoking. Even if you are a non-smoker and teetotal, working or socialising in a smoky or dry atmosphere will affect your voice. Other voice changes are part of the natural life cycle. Our voices change as we age. Women may notice a difference in their voice following hormonal changes during pregnancy, menstruation, or the menopause.

Learning to listen to your voice will help you to develop an awareness of when it needs greater attention. You need to be particularly alert to any changes in your physical health, such as infections from colds and coughs. Voice difficulties may also arise as a side-effect of certain medications or as a consequence of an allergy. Your psychological state is also important. Stress and other emotional concerns sometimes manifest themselves in a voice problem. Finally you need to pay attention to your diet. Some spicy foods are irritating, and indigestion caused by irregular or late night meals can affect the voice. Sometimes we are guilty of voluntarily abusing our voices, such as prolonged shouting at a football match or screaming at pop concert.

Making a presentation involves using the voice for an extended period of time. In addition to this, anxiety can make it difficult to relax, which also has an adverse affect on voice quality. Here are some quick tips on how the presenter can care for the voice:

✧ Prevention is better than cure

Eat a balanced diet and keep regular mealtimes. Carry out a programme of practical voice exercises. (See the section at the end.)

The night before your presentation:

- Get enough sleep
- Avoid excesses of alcohol and smoking
- Avoid eating a heavy or spicy meal near bedtime.

✧ Work with your environment

- Check out the acoustics before your presentation; if in doubt, use amplification
- Open windows to keep the room well ventilated

- Have a jar of still water ready to drink during the presentation. But consume in moderation!

⬦ **Take control of your body**

- Relax. You are going to enjoy yourself!
- Start with a smile; this will help relax the jaw area.
- Look round at the audience and not down at your notes
- Check your posture. Is it symmetrical and balanced? Maintain a calm breathing pattern using the diaphragm.

⬦ **Vocal tips**

- Do not force your voice
- Sip water or swallow if you develop a nervous cough or want to clear your throat
- Do not try to talk over extraneous noises. (Turn the overhead off, ask people to listen if they are talking.)

⬦ **Conserve your voice**

You do not have to talk all the time. Conserve your voice by decreasing the amount of time you do the talking. The audience can ask questions, watch a video or look at an overhead.

Avoid increasing volume to get attention. Use intonation, pauses and a change in pace to gain the interest of the audience.

It is particularly important to care for your voice if you have had a cold, cough or other infection. Remember stress and other adverse psychological states affect the voice.

Use the self-monitoring checklist to identify problems at an early stage.

Self-monitoring checklist

Watch out for the signs that your voice needs a rest.
Listen to the sound of your voice:

- Is it croaky or hoarse?
- Does it sound weak?
- Have you recently developed problems in maintaining a note whilst singing?
- Have you lost your voice altogether?

Think about how your voice 'feels':
- ◦ Is your throat tight or tense?
- ◦ Is your throat sore?
- ◦ Does your voice feel tired?
- ◦ Do you feel you are straining to make yourself heard?
- ◦ Are you forcing your voice?

Listen to what your friends and family are saying:
- ◦ 'You are always shouting?'
- ◦ 'You sound as if you have a cold?'
- ◦ 'You sound really tense.'
- ◦ 'Are you tired? Your voice sounds croaky.'

Everybody has odd days when their voice is not at its best. These are usually due to isolated events such as hormonal changes or overindulgence of food and alcohol the night before. Sometimes however, these are signs of an ongoing problem. See your doctor immediately if you have any concerns regarding your voice. They will be able to refer you for specialist advice.

Practical exercises for effective use of voice

The exercises in this section will help you to develop the posture, breathing patterns, resonance and articulatory control that will enable you to use your voice effectively. They can be used to prepare for an important presentation or as a general programme to maintain good voice patterns. Remember 'good habits become unconscious' (Bunch 1982). The exercises are divided into six categories:

    R Relaxation

    H&N Head and Neck

    B Breathing

    Re Resonance

    A Articulatory Awareness

    E Expressiveness

Some authors suggest that a programme to train the voice should be carried out every day, starting several weeks before the presentation. This is the ideal situation. In reality this may be difficult or impossible. Each individual has to work out a programme that meets their needs and accommodates the demands of life.

In general, it is a good idea to start well ahead of the date of your talk, and to have frequent but regular sessions. Choose at least one exercise from *each* category to form your programme for a session. Exercises should be carried out in the order of the categories below, i.e. starting with relaxation, moving on to head and neck and so on. Add interest by varying your exercises. If you have extra time, choose additional relaxation and breathing ones.

A typical example of a session programme might be:

Relaxation
Visualisation

Head and Neck
Shoulder hunches

Breathing
Sustaining an 'S' on one breath

Resonance
Alternating between an oral sound and a nasal sound

Articulation
Saying tongue twisters aloud

Intonation
Saying tongue twisters using different emotional tones.

N.B. Always consult your G.P. before starting the exercises if you have any neck, back or other physical problems.

Positioning
Before you start the exercises make sure you are comfortable. Find a spacious area where you are free from interruptions and the atmosphere is warm and pleasant. You may find a slightly darkened room is better. Some exercises require you to lie down, while others are best carried out in a standing or sitting position. Some exercises are suitable for a variety of postures, and you may want to try alternating between lying down, sitting and standing.

Lying down

Place a mat on the floor. Lie down on your back with knees bent. Let your arms rest at the side of your body. Spread your shoulders out so that they are resting on the floor, and not raised up. (This position can also be tried by lying on a firm bed or couch.)

Standing

Stand with your feet placed apart so that they are in line with your hips and pointing forwards. Let your arms hang loosely at your sides. Stand tall. Imagine a wire is coming out of the crown of your head. It is pulling you gently up, as if you were suspended from the ceiling. Remember the wire is pulling you gently. Shoulders should be back and down in a relaxed position. Your head facing forwards, not tilting back or drooping forwards or cocked to one side.

Sitting

Straight backed chairs with no arm rests are suitable for this position. Check the height. You need one that allows you easily to place both feet flat on the floor. Sit in the chair with legs slightly apart. Do not allow yourself to slump. Imagine a wire is coming out of the crown of your head. It is pulling you gently up, as if you were suspended from the ceiling. Remember the wire is pulling you gently. Shoulders should be back and down in a relaxed position. Your head facing forwards, not tilting back or drooping forwards or cocked to one side.

✧ R Relaxation

Relaxation is central to all the other exercises in this section and should always be first in your programme.

Hint – You may like to record the italicised script in the first exercise onto a cassette for your own relaxation tape.

R This exercise will help you to recognise the difference between a state of relaxation and a state of tension. You start with your toes and work up through the body to the head.

(1) *Scrunch up your toes as hard as you can.* The muscles in your toes and feet will tense up. Can you feel tension any where else? Maybe in the feet, the ankles or the calves? You will probably be able to feel the tension of contracting muscles in all these places. You can see how tension is never isolated to one part of the body.

Now relax your toes. Stretch them out. Give them a wiggle! Shake off the stress like droplets of water. Circle your ankles. First clockwise. Then anti-clockwise. Let the tension flow out of your feet. Check your feet are flat on the floor before starting the next bit.

(2) *Tense the muscles of your calves.* Can you do it without contracting any other muscle? Actually it is impossible. Think about where you can feel tension. Is it in your ankles, in your thighs or in your knees? What has happened to your feet? They have probably been raised off the floor slightly. *Now gently let your calf muscles relax. Check your feet are flat on the floor. You may want to give your toes a little wiggle again. Let your legs go very heavy, like lead. Rest your legs there, as if you have no control over their movement.*

(3) *Next, tense the muscles of the thighs.* Pretend you are holding an imaginary orange between them. Careful, you might drop it. *Keep squeezing tightly. Hold. Hold. Hold.* Can you feel where else your legs are tense? Do not forget to breathe.

Then gently relax the muscles. Slowly easing out the tension from your thighs, your calves, until it ebbs out of your feet. Check your feet are flat on the floor again.

(4) *Tighten your tummy muscles. Make it hard like a wall. Hold for a few moments, then slowly relax. Repeat using the muscles of your buttocks. Squeeze them together. Hold for a few moments, then slowly relax.*

(5) We now move up the body to the hands. (Remember your hands and arms should have been resting at your sides during the previous exercises.) *Clench your fists as hard as you can.* Feel the tension stretching up your arms. Can you feel any tension around the jaw area? *Hold this position for a few seconds, then slowly relax. Still keeping your hands in a fist shape, gradually uncurl your fingers. Shake your hands. Let them flop at the wrist. Then return your arms to the side.*

(6) *Squeeze the inside of your arms against the sides of your chest.* Feel the tension across your chest. *Then relax your arms and chest. Finish with a gentle sigh.*

(7) The final part of the exercise is for the head and neck. Check your head is in the midline facing forwards, no tilting backwards or

dropping forwards. *Gently drop your chin down towards your chest.* (Do not force it to touch your chest.) *Let it rest there for a few moments.* Feel the tension in the back of the neck. *Then slowly lift your head until you are looking straight ahead again.* Avoid leading with your chin.

Now gently let your head tilt backwards so you are looking at the ceiling. Feel the muscles in your throat stretching. *Stay in that position for a few moments. Then gently bring your head forwards until it is resting in the midline again.*

(8) *Let your head rest gently forward. Close your eyes.* Breathe gently. *Feel your whole body relaxing.* Finally, slowly raise your head up to the midline.

This exercise should have given you a good idea of how it feels when your body is tense and when it is relaxed. You will also have learned how the tension passes from one area to another. If you feel tension forming in any part of your body you can start to concentrate on releasing that tension and relaxing.

R Sometimes the body needs re-energising. Try this exercise to wake yourself up. Stand tall with your shoulders back and down in relaxed position. (Avoid pulling your shoulders back.) Slowly raise one arm above your head and then the other. Stretch them up to the ceiling. Hold the position for a moment, and then slowly open your arms outward. Stretch them out to the side and then slowly lower them. Follow the stretches with some gentle shaking of the hands and then the feet. Alternatively try some circling movements. Complete the exercise by lightly slapping your back and shoulder area to get the blood moving about.

R Visualisation is a technique often used to help people relax. It is a simple idea and works by encouraging people to have nice thoughts. You may like to try this exercise at the end of the first exercise while you have your eyes closed. All you have to do is think of a pleasant experience. For some people this may be lying on a beach. Picture yourself stretched out on the sand. Try to think about all the sounds you might hear. A seagull, waves against the shoreline, the quietness compared with a noisy street. What sensations might you feel? The heat of the sun against your skin, sand draining through your fingertips. Do not forget the smells and taste. Sun tan lotion, saltwater on the lips, a cooling ice-lolly. Spend a few minutes concentrating on these thoughts. Feeling totally relaxed.

R Visualisation can be more specific. Think about your presentation. Your delivery is faultless. Your audio-visual aids work perfectly. The audience are enthusiastic. You feel great. Concentrate on that warm feeling of success. Savour the moment. This will help build up your confidence for your presentation.

✧ H&N Head and Neck

As the head and neck area is very important to voice production it merits a section of its own. The exercises will help you explore some of the tension specific to this area and help you release the strain of tense muscles.

Hint – Stand or sit squarely with your shoulders straight but relaxed. Start all of these exercises with your head in the midline so that it is not tilted to one side, backwards or drooping forward.

H&N Hunch your shoulders so that they are almost touching your ears. Feel all the tension in your neck. Then drop the shoulders back down. This should be a dropping movement. The shoulders should not be forced down or pulled sharply. A friend can help here by checking that your shoulders are down and not raised up by standing behind you with their hands on your shoulders. Repeat this exercise five times.

H&N Gently circle your shoulders. First with a backwards movement and then with a forwards movement. Repeat, but this time rotate one shoulder then the other.

H&N Gently turn your head to the right and then return it to the midline. Repeat the exercise to the left. As you do this exercise feel the tension in the side that is stretched in the turn. Repeat the exercise five times.

H&N Look to the left so that your chin is near your left shoulder. Drop your chin. This should be a comfortable position. Stop if you feel pain or pulling. Gently roll your head round to the right shoulder. Imagine you are looking at a ball rolling from one side of your lap to the other. Imagine your head is a giant ball bearing. Very heavy. So heavy it is impossible to lift it. Allow it to slowly roll. Gently roll your head to the midline and raise your head. Repeat for the right side.

H&N You will need to stand or sit up for this exercise. Stand straight and hold your arms out at the side. Aim to keep them at shoulder height – no lower and no higher. Slowly circle your hands as if you were drawing a small circle in the air with your fingertips. Do ten circles in a forwards direction and then ten in a backwards direction. Next swing both arms to the right side of the body. Your left arm will have to cross over the front of the body. Now swing both arms round to the left. Your right arm will have to cross over the front of your body.

✧ B Breathing

Start each exercise with a relaxed pattern of breathing. Place your hands on your diaphragm or middle, so that your hands are flat and the tips of your fingers are touching. Breathe in slowly through the nose. Notice how the fingers are pushed apart as you fill your lungs. (Do not push your stomach out to make this happen.) It is just like a balloon filling with air. When you are ready, slowly expel the air through the mouth in a long gentle stream. Your finger tips should gently start to meet as your middle starts to flatten. Wait until you need to fill with air again. Then slowly breathe in and out as above. Once you are happy with this pattern of breathing you can start the exercises.

B As you breathe out make a long sighing sound. Concentrate on the feeling in your middle. Next try a long 's' sound, like a tyre deflating. (Remember to take a breath between exercises.) Do not force the sound. Let it gently out. Count to yourself to see how long you can sustain it. Try starting quietly and gradually increase the volume. Then start with a loud 's' and let it gradually get quieter. Experiment with making lots of short 's' sounds. Try a sequence with some quiet ones interspersed with some loud ones.

B As you breathe out make different rhythmic patterns using the sound 's'. Try:

loud (S) and quiet (s)

s s S s s S s s

long (s _____) and short (s __)

s__ s _____ s __ s __ s __ s _____ s __ s __

noise and silence

sss   sss   sss

Aim to make the sounds on one breath.

B As you breathe out make a long sighing sound. Concentrate on the area around your diaphragm. As you sigh gently make an 'ah' sound. It should sound almost like a 'haaah'. Repeat this several times. Try using different vowel sounds – oo, ee, I, oh, a.

B As you breathe out make a vowel sound. Start with 'oo'. Repeat the sound several times using one breath. If you are lying down imagine you are propelling the sound up to the ceiling. If you are sitting or standing imagine you are propelling the sound towards a distant wall or out of the window. Think about the sound coming from the diaphragm. Do not push at it from your vocal folds. Repeat using other vowel sounds.

✧ Re Resonance

These exercises use a tactile and auditory approach to improving resonance. So you feel and hear the resonance in your voice.

Hint – Experiment with different pitch levels using an 'ah' sound, going from a high note down to a low note. Find a level that feels comfortable and sounds good. This is your optimum pitch level and will provide you with the best resonance.

Re Gently hum. How long can you sustain the sound? Can you feel your lips and teeth vibrating? If not, try saying 'm' several times before trying a long hum. When you are comfortable with producing a hum, place your finger tips on the sides of your nose to feel the vibrations. Then drop your hands to your cheeks. Can you feel the vibrations? Try altering your pitch so that it rises and falls.

Re Open your mouth and let your jaw relax. Place the tip of your tongue behind your bottom teeth. Say the sound that occurs at the end of the word 'sung'. This relies on resonance from the nasal cavity. Once you are able to produce this sound, alternate with the sound 'ah'. This sound relies on resonance in the oral cavity. Practise moving from one sound to the other; from nasal to oral resonance. Think about the sounds being forward in the mouth.

Re Try saying this sequence of words. 'hook hawk hock hut herd had head hey hid heed' Feel how the tongue moves from the back of the mouth to the front. Compare the shape of your lips for the word hook with the words had and heed.

Re Try yawning and vocalising at the same time. You can use nonsense syllables or short phrases with two or three words. The yawning should help to relax the muscles in your face and improve your resonance.

✧ A Articulatory Awareness

These exercises will increase your awareness of articulatory movements. They will help you to increase the precision of movement required for making speech sounds.

Hint – Use a hand mirror to check how you are doing with these lip and tongue exercises.

A Feel around the inside of your mouth using the tip of your tongue. Run it around the edge of your teeth, then feel the inside and the outside of them. Stick it out as far as you can and then waggle it from side to side. Then lick around your lips clockwise then anti clockwise. Touch your top lip with your tongue tip and then your bottom lip. Try singing la-la-la at the same time.

A Practise saying these three sounds together.

P T K

How fast can you say them without making a mistake? Avoid adding a vowel. So you say p rather than pea or per. Try:

pppp tttt kkkk

Now say the sequence backwards.

K T P

kkkk tttt pppp

A Say some tongue twisters aloud. Try to speed up without making a mistake or slurring the sounds.

A Place a finger between the teeth and say the following vowel sounds:

ah

ee

oh

or

oo

Now remove your finger and repeat the exercise. Aim to keep your mouth as open as possible. Read a passage keeping the same open mouth position.

A Choose one list of words and phrases. Read them aloud as fast as you can without making a mistake.

A	B
pattercake	peppermint
bail of paper	biscuit bowl
teapot	tall and dark
docker	departure
caterpillar	coffee maker
shopkeeper	shooter
scissors	sizzling sausages
zodiac sign	zoo keeper
chocolate	cheesecake
bake me an apple pie	teddy bear's tea party

C	D
buttercups	peanut butter
tea towel	tuppence
dirty duck	dandelion tea
cornucopia	candy floss
garden gate	guinea pig
shortcake	cheroots
seven sons	sandwich
zigzag	zither
cherry pie	chariots
shut the garden gate	sweeping past the strawberries

✧ **E Expressiveness**

Variations in intonation patterns, pitch, pace and volume gives the voice variety and adds interest. These exercises provide practice in using the voice expressively.

Hint – tape record yourself or get feedback from friends on how accurate you are in expressing different feelings with your voice. Record a sentence or a passage and then leave a pause before you state the appropriate emotion. You can test yourself by listening to the tape and trying to guess the feeling. Wind on the tape to find the answer you previously recorded.

E Choose a short sentence and say it in a variety of ways. Listen to how the tone of the voice changes the meaning.

For example:

'I love you' (why don't you love me?)

'I love you' (how many more times do I have to say it?)

'I love you' (for always and forever)

'I love you' (is that what you are saying?)

'I love you' (you sexy thing)

'I love you' (I can't live without you)

'I love you' (Please, don't go)

'I love you' (you're such a cutie!)

E Choose a short passage from a novel, a newspaper or a magazine. Re-write the passage, keeping phrase groups to one line. Practise reading it aloud pausing at the end of a phrase group. It may help if you beat out the rhythm with your hand.

E Choose a short piece from the newspaper. Read it aloud using a different tone of voice each time. Use your voice to express envy, disbelief, enthusiasm, sarcasm, and concern.

E Give a short command in a variety of emotional tones.

For example: 'Come in' as if you are angry. Try the following tones:

You are sad

You are shy

You are exasperated

You are surprised

You are depressed

You are elated

You are frightened

You are confidant.

E Collect together some old greeting cards. Try to include ones with a variety of messages – birthday, retirement, birth, moving home, thank you, bereavement, and seasonal. Read aloud the messages using the appropriate tone to convey congratulations, commiseration, love or pleasure.

E Notice how the significance of words is altered in this sentence when the emphasis shifts from one word to another.

- Jack is coming to *Fiona's* party (not Jane's party)
- *Jack* is coming to Fiona's party (not David)
- Jack is coming to Fiona's *party* (not the church service)
- Jack *is* coming to Fiona's party (I thought he couldn't make it)

Find other sentences and experiment by placing the emphasis on different words.

E Practise reciting poetry. Use intonation and tone of voice to add interest and express different emotions. Try reading a funny poem with a serious tone or a love poem in an angry voice.

Summary Points

- Keep a relaxed and open posture.
- Breathe from the diaphragm, and not the shoulders. Take breaths when you need them. Remember to breathe out.
- Look at the audience. This will keep your head in the midline and help projection and audibility.
- Help project your voice by speaking to the people in the back row, and using resonance.
- Increase the clarity of your voice by using distinct articulation, and slowing down the rate of your speech. Keeping to the natural rhythm of your speech and avoid exaggerating your words.
- Use your voice to express yourself. Vary your pitch and intonation to make your voice more interesting.
- Use silence for dramatic effect. Pausing can add emphasis and draw attention to an important point.

Delivering Content

By the time you are ready to do your presentation the content of your talk will be as familiar to you as your name and address. Your main concern is not 'what is your message' but 'getting your message across' to your audience. This section looks at the ways in which you can communicate your content more effectively.

✧ Choose your words carefully

In every presentation there will be a certain amount of assumed knowledge. You will have expectations about what the audience know and understand about procedures, terminology, or medical details. Your research on the background and experience of the audience will have helped you to determine your choice of vocabulary and the complexity of your language. If you misjudge this assumed knowledge you will easily lose your audience in over complex explanations. In general it is better to avoid jargon and abbreviations.

✧ Make it clear

Deliver a clear message. Avoid sentence constructions or words that are confusing or lack impact. To make your speech clearer remember to:

- ○ Use active not passive sentences. 'Regular brushing reduces tooth decay' is better than 'tooth decay is reduced by regular brushing.'

- ○ Avoid ambiguous words. For example, homonyms (words that sound the same but differ in meaning), are more difficult to differentiate in spoken communication as there are no cues from spelling.

- ○ Re-phrase ambiguous questions or statements. For example, the question 'Where did you have the X-ray?' may mean where is the x-ray department or which part of your body was x-rayed.

- Use simple sentences. They are always preferable to complex ones, regardless of the intellectual ability of your audience.

- Put the most important piece of information at the beginning of the sentence. Look at the example below. Which of the statements is clearer? Place a piece of paper over the sentences, with a hole large enough to see one word at a time. This will simulate how you receive information when you are listening as opposed to reading. (You are not able to see the words that have gone before or the words that are about to be said.)

> Cerebral palsy, cleft palate, Down's Syndrome are all associated with hearing loss.

> Hearing loss is associated with cerebral palsy, cleft palate, Down's Syndrome.

✧ Be fluent

Cut out verbal fillers like 'well', 'um', 'okay then', 'what's next'. Too many hesitations make it difficult for the audience to assimilate information, and the presentation becomes disjointed. Waffle makes your communication less effective. Look at the following example:

The audience's attention increases slightly just before a demonstration, video or other audio-visual aid. This is due to the effects of anticipation, change of stimulus and the natural pause that occurs. Look at how this presenter loses the opportunity to use the time to make an important point by filling the pause with waffle. 'Ah. I see. It's OK. This is the machine we have in our department. There are so many different models. I have used other machines myself. They are all quite similar really. Right, I'll just switch it on and show you this overhead'.

✧ Use words to structure your presentation

The audience need to have a general understanding of the direction in which you are leading them. In your introduction you will have told your audience the purpose of your presentation and given a brief outline. You will need to give further orientating information throughout your talk.

Use specific words and phrases to alert the audience to key points in your presentation (Brown 1982). Phrases like 'The fundamental issue...' 'The primary consideration...' or 'This is a very important point...' help the audience to identify the main points. However, be careful not to overdo it. A friend who recently attended a computer course was left bemused by the multitude of important points. The presenter had introduced nearly every item with 'This is very important'.

At the end of each section summarise the main points to indicate to the audience that you have finished a section. Start the next topic with a few introductory sentences. For instance, 'We have looked at the benefits of a computerised appointments system. These include faster access to information, multi-user access and reduced staffing costs. Let's now look at how such a system might be implemented.'

✧ Choose words with impact

Forsyth (1995) suggests using words with impact. Think about the words you use in your presentation. Are they powerful and imaginative? Or bland, everyday words? The word 'nice' is commonplace but lacks power. It has many meanings including pleasant, cultured, and affable. Compare 'The presenter was nice.' with these sentences:

'The presenter was considerate'

'The presenter was friendly'

'The presenter was excellent'

The meanings are much more precise, and therefore the word has more impact. Use impact words to get your message across.

✧ Be natural

Never adopt an unfamiliar accent or attempt to dramatise your performance. Use your own 'voice' when speaking. You will sound natural and more relaxed.

✧ Use spoken english

Spoken English has a different grammatical form from written English. It has a less formal style and structure. This is partly why reading from a script in a presentation often sounds stilted. A script uses the written form rather than the spoken. Written scripts are a definite no-no for presenters.

✧ Pace your delivery to suit the audience

The presenter controls the rate that information is supplied to the listener. This rate will depend on the type of material, the nature of the audience and the familiarity of terminology. Remember complex or unfamiliar material takes longer to assimilate and therefore needs a slower delivery. The pace of a presentation can be controlled through the adept use of pauses, repetition and audio-visual aids. For example, mask out points on your overhead by covering them with paper, until you are ready to present them.

Sometimes the delivery can be too slow. This is because the listener can process the spoken word faster than the rate speech is produced (Armstrong 1984). The audience can easily become bored and lose concentration if the delivery is too slow. Use changes in rhythm and intonation to add interest to your speech. Present complex material quickly in the form of visual images.

✧ Use silence

Silence can be used for dramatic effect. Newscasters often pause before announcing a serious news item or major disaster. This signals to the audience the gravity and importance of the message. A pause at the beginning or end of an important point will give it emphasis (Freeburn 1993). Pausing at the end of an explanation or example allows the audience time to assimilate information.

✧ Dealing with questions

When and how you take questions will depend on the nature of the presentation and the size of the audience. Check with the organisers on how questions are to be handled. Is there a slot at the end? Is it appropriate to take questions during the talk? Is there a chair person?

The type of questions asked by your audience will provide you with information on their attitudes, their knowledge base, and their interests. Use the audience's responses to monitor how much the audience are under-standing of the topic.

When you are asked a question remember:

- To listen. Wait until the questioner has stopped talking, before you start thinking about how to frame your response.
- To ask for a repetition if the question is unclear.
- To speak to the whole audience and not just the questioner.
- To keep your responses brief and to the point.
- To relate your reply to the topic. Do not allow yourself to get side-tracked onto someone's pet subject.

Sometimes you may not know the answer. Do not be afraid to admit it. It is impossible for one person to know all the answers. You can always throw the question out to the whole audience to discuss.

Keep control of question time by making the boundaries clear. Tell the audience when you are expecting questions, and set a limit on the number to be asked. Bear in mind that too many questions can upset your timing, and make it difficult for people to follow the thread of the discussion.

You may need to delay your response to a question, if it interrupts an explanation or it is out of context. Acknowledge the question and explain that you will deal with it later. For example, 'That is a very pertinent point. I would like to come back to that after the session on planning, which has some information relevant to your question. Is that OK?'

When taking questions indicate to whom you will respond and in what order. It is useful both to yourself and the rest of the audience if questioners identify themselves by name and occupation before speaking. In a workshop this is a quick way for people to learn names and find out about each other. It also puts you on an equal footing with audience. You will now know their names and occupations.

Difficult questions can arise for a number of reasons. The questioner may have their own personal agenda. They may object to your statements or be using the question to demonstrate their own 'superior' knowledge. Try to stay calm and remain unemotional. A few deep breaths before responding will help. Always acknowledge the questioner and the question, and then try one of the following responses.

An objection hidden in a question

Bring the objection out into the open. Here is an example – 'Doesn't all this advice on feeding and caring for babies make parents too reliant on health visitors. At quite a cost I might add.' The underlying objection in this question is cost, and possibly the issue of de-skilling parents. The presenter needs to explain the benefits of regular contact with a health visitor, and the cost effectiveness of early screening and health promotion.

The questioner has completely missed the point

The rest of the audience are likely to look embarrassed as the questioner demonstrates their stupidity. As a presenter you need to bring the questioner gently back to the topic. You can take the blame by saying 'Sorry I seem to have misled you here. What I actually meant was...'

The verbose questioner

Try to identify the main question and respond to this. You may have to halt the flow by using non-verbal cues. Indicate that you are about to respond by nodding your head several times, moving away from the questioner and dropping eye-contact. If necessary, hold up your hands in a 'stop' gesture.

Several questions in one

Either deal with the first or main question, or respond to each one in turn if you have time.

Attempts to sidetrack the issue

An example would be 'this is all very well but the important or interesting question here is...' Acknowledge that it is an interesting point, but remind the questioner politely what you are there to talk about. Suggest that you talk together after the presentation.

The muddled questioner

It is very unclear what this questioner is actually asking. (The audience will usually have bemused looks too.) Check you have understood the question – 'So what you want to know is... Have I got it right?'. Re-phrase the question before answering so that it is clear for the rest of the audience.

Attempts to demonstrate superior knowledge by a self-appointed expert

Never try to bluff your way through if you are unsure of the answer. If not, throw the question out to other members of the audience. Alternatively ask the questioner what they think. They will probably be only too willing to tell you.

Try to anticipate any questions or criticisms in your preparation and decide upon your responses.

✧ Support the spoken word

Help the audience to understand the spoken message by supporting it with visual and auditory images, the written word and body language. This means using your audio-visual aids, supplying appropriate hand-outs and using gesture, body posture and facial expression to supplement the spoken word. Look at the sections on 'Using Non-Verbal Communication' and 'Preparation' for more ideas.

✧ Use hand-outs

Most presentations benefit from the support of written handouts. They are one way of helping the audience to understand and remember your message. Types of hand-out include:

- A complete transcript of the presentation
- A partial transcript that gives a summary of the main points

- ○ Gapped hand-outs that are completed as part of the lecture; for example, labelling a diagram
- ○ A list of references
- ○ A list of suggested reading
- ○ A glossary of terms
- ○ Copies of tables, diagrams, or graphs
- ○ Copies of overheads
- ○ Instructions for activities.

Your choice of hand-out will be dictated by the purpose of your presentation and the nature of the audience. A conference organiser may request a complete transcript, whereas gapped handouts are appropriate for an undergraduate lecture.

Make a decision about when to give out the hand-outs. Do they need to refer to them during your talk? Will they distract the listener? Distributing paper to a large group can be time-consuming and disrupt the flow of the presentation. Place hand-outs on chairs before the audience arrive, or leave them at the back of the room for people to collect as they leave. Tell the audience the hand-outs you will be supplying, especially if they are expected to take notes.

Summary Points

- ○ Choose your words carefully, and match your vocabulary and language level to your audience. Use words that have impact.
- ○ Make sure your message is clear. Avoid any ambiguous words, jargon, or abbreviations. Use simple, clear sentences.
- ○ Be fluent by cutting out waffle and reducing hesitations.
- ○ Provide the audience with verbal indicators of the structure of your talk by summarising at the end of a section and introducing new topics.
- ○ Avoid reading from a script.
- ○ Match the pace of delivery to the complexity of the task. Complex tasks need a slower delivery with more explanation.

- Use pauses to add emphasis, interest and to give the audience time to assimilate information.

- Use the audience's responses to questions to gauge their level of knowledge, understanding, and attitudes.

- Respond to questions briefly and clearly. Relate the information back to the topic.

- Set up rules about how and when you will respond to questions. Prepare responses to possible objections or queries.

- Support the spoken word with audio-visual aids, hand-outs and non-verbal communication.

- Help your audience to understand and remember your message by providing hand-outs.

19

Establishing Rapport with the Audience

Scene setting

Establishing rapport with your audience starts from the moment you begin your talk, if not before. As you walk in front of the audience, your appearance and body language will send out signals. The audience will unconsciously be making judgements about your personality, expertise and background. So approach the presentation with a confident and open manner.

Introductions are a brief but essential beginning to your presentation. It gives the audience time to focus, and it lets them know something about you. Remember to tell the audience your name, title and some details about where you work. This may seem an obvious statement but these details can easily be forgotten. It is also useful to emphasise the factors that give you credibility on the subject of the presentation.

After your introduction provide an outline of your presentation. State the purpose of your talk and give a brief overview of the content. These details can also be displayed on an overhead at the same time. Remind the audience about the proposed length of your session, and when refreshment breaks will be taken.

The audience will feel more comfortable if they know something about what is expected of them. Will they be actively involved? When can they ask questions? It may be appropriate at this point to have a question and answer session to help structure the presentation to their specific needs.

Engaging the audience

Eye-contact

When we want to speak to another person we usually make eye-contact with them first. Unless you are speaking on the radio, effective communication with an audience involves making and keeping eye-contact. How much do you look at your audience? How do you feel? Comfortable or self-conscious?

You may need to make a deliberate effort to look at the audience. Focus on individuals who are smiling or look interested. Remember to glance around at the whole audience from time to time, even those at the back and to the side. First impressions are lasting, so start off by looking at your audience. Memorise your opening comments so you are able to look around at the audience.

Stimulation

Get your audience interested right from the start. Here is an example of an unusual introduction to a lecture on psychology presented at a career's conference. The speaker was interrupted by a police officer chasing a man through the lecture hall. A few minutes later the officer returned and asked members of the audience for a description of the suspect. Some people described him as tall with brown hair, others as short with black hair. A few people were unsure whether it was a man or a woman. In fact, it was a set up to demonstrate to the audience the unreliability of witness observations. It was a very successful and stimulating way of introducing students to why we study memory. You may want to think of less dramatic ways of introducing your subject! The above example worked well because it was novel, the audience were actively involved, it was unexpected, and it used a very practical example. It was also pitched at just the right level for an audience of sixth formers.

Participation

You are more likely to establish a rapport with an audience who are involved in your presentation. In an informal talk you can encourage questions at the end of each section. This will help to clarify any misunderstandings and provide you with feedback. Find out the audience's viewpoint on issues, and ask for contributions from individuals with relevant experience. In a formal setting, or with a very large audience use rhetorical questions to provoke reflection, and to act as an introduction to your next topic. For example, in a lecture on incontinence, the question 'How does the body know when the bladder is full?' introduces the topic of the nervous system.

Help the audience to relate items to their own experience. A lecturer giving a talk on how animals attract a mate introduced the topic to her audience by asking them to think about what attracted them to their partners. This was a fun exercise that got everyone chatting.

Audience feedback

Get feedback from the audience on how well you are getting across your message. Do they seem interested and amused by your examples? Have they been stimulated to ask questions? Check for signs of boredom, confusion, or annoyance.

Remember:

- **Watch** – facial expression and posture
- **Listen** – Are they fidgeting? Are papers being rustled? Are people talking to each other?
- **Ask for feedback** – Is that clear? Would you like more examples? Tell me if I am going too fast or too slow? Ask questions to check how well they are following.

Delivery

An audience who have to work at understanding the message will soon lose interest. Their requirements will influence your choice of language and examples, and alter the emphasis of your talk (Freeburn 1993). Modify your pace, style of delivery and speech to suit their needs, and avoid jargon or complicated expressions that people will find difficult.

Use your language to build a bridge between you and the audience. Forsyth (1995) advises caution when using personal pronouns. Statements that begin 'You should…' and 'I think you…' are to be avoided. Substitute 'we' if possible, so 'you should take a thorough case history' becomes 'we know that a thorough case history is essential'.

The manner of your delivery is just as important as the content. If you are enthusiastic about your talk, your audience will be enthusiastic. If you believe in what you are saying, your audience will believe in you. Never feel that you have to prove your superiority. This is the quickest way of getting people's backs up. You are there because you have something to say that is of interest to those present; not because you are better than them.

Shared agenda

Your talk needs to be relevant and of interest to the audience. There must be a shared agenda, and your audience must be aware that this exists. The point of contact may be a shared interest; a joint responsibility; or mutual goals. Shimoda (1994) describes the audience as a partner in the presentation. Try to relate your experience and skills to those of the audience, for example 'as nurses we often have to deal with bereavement'. The implied message is that the presenter shares the same occupation and has had the same experiences. This is where a thorough preparation is important. You need to know your audience before you can share ideas.

Time-keeping

The audience will appreciate good time-keeping. Aim to start and finish on time. You will find tips on how to plan your presentation within the allotted time in the section on 'Preparation'.

Final point

Make time to summarise your main points at the end of the talk. Aim to finish your talk with one single message the audience can take away with them.

Memorise your final comments and remember to look round at the audience as you say them. Do not feel embarrassed to acknowledge any applause or appreciative comments. You may feel a great relief that your ordeal is over, but try not to sag before you get back to your seat.

Action Points

(1) Think of presentations where you have felt no rapport for the presenter. My list includes:

- The speaker was too quiet (national conference)

- The speaker made it very clear that he had better things to do with his time (undergraduate lecture)

- Inappropriate remarks – sexist, racist, or plain insensitivity (various lectures)

- Failure to recognise pace of delivery and amount of information was inappropriate for the audience(post-graduate course)

- Not knowing the audience(safety at work lecture for female health workers. Speaker assumed all the women present were nurses based on hospital wards)

- Lack of preparation. Speaker hand wrote overheads during talk (in-service study day).

(2) Think about speakers whom you felt established a good rapport with the audience. My list includes:

- An interesting presentation (the rules governing the use of English speech sounds explained in terms of a chess game)

- The presenter had a charming personality. This is difficult to define! (neurology consultant speaking to undergraduates)

- Presenter started with a self-effacing comment (well-known politician about his lack of technical expertise at a conference on IT. This struck a chord with many of the audience.)

- An account of working life using numerous witty anecdotes (well-known public figure at a graduation ceremony).

Summary Points

- Establishing rapport starts from the first moment of your talk.

- Set the scene for your presentation by introducing yourself clearly, stating your objectives and outlining your talk. Explain the format of the presentation.

- Remember to look at your audience. Concentrate on individuals but also glance round at the whole audience.

- Make your topic interesting and relevant for the audience. Start with something that captures their attention.

- Encourage the audience to participate by using questions and asking for contributions.

- Regularly check the audience's understanding and interest in the topic by looking at their body language.

- Do not allow your language to become a barrier between you and the audience. Avoid jargon.

- Use your language to build a bridge between you and the audience. Avoid starting statements with 'you should'. Use 'we' instead.

- A successful presentation is one where the presenter and the audience share the same agenda. Find out what interests, goals or responsibilities you share with your audience.

- Good time-keeping is crucial.

- Leave time at the end to give a summary of the main points. Memorise your closing remarks.

20

Using Non-Verbal Communication

Non-verbal communication is about the messages that are conveyed by the movements and position of our limbs, facial features and body. This is popularly known as body language. In a presentation the following behaviours are important:

- eye-contact
- facial expression
- gestures
- posture
- position
- orientation.

You can use non-verbal communication in several ways during your presentation.

- Use it to support your verbal message.
- Use it to add interest and enliven your talk.
- Use it to establish rapport with the audience.
- Use it as an alternative way of communicating your message.
- Use it to help interaction with the audience.
- Use the audience's non-verbal behaviour for feedback on how your talk is received.

Below is a description of how each behaviour might contribute to your presentation.

Eye-contact

You need to look at your audience. This helps to build a rapport by making the audience feel you are interested in them. Eye-contact also helps to maintain attention and interest. A lack of eye-contact will suggest that you are nervous or insincere. If you are continually glancing at your notes, you will also seem unprepared.

Eye-contact allows you to get feedback from the audience. You can see how they are reacting to your talk. Watch their faces and posture to gauge their level of understanding, interest and involvement. (Look at eye-contact in the chapter on *Establishing Rapport with the Audience* for more ideas.)

Facial expression

The face is the most important non-verbal channel. It is capable of very fine movements and is extremely mobile. These various changes in expression enable us to express our feelings and to signal different attitudes. Specific movements of the face are also linked with speech (Trower *et al.* 1978). For example, a frown might accompany 'I'm not clear about this'.

It is important to match your facial expression to your verbal message. Are you sending mixed messages? Does your facial expression correspond with your tone of voice? Show your enthusiasm in your face, as well as by your tone of voice. The audience is more likely to believe what they see than what they hear (Zaidel and Mehrabian 1969).

Remember anxiety or concentration may unconsciously be revealed in your facial features, so you need to monitor your expression. This does not mean putting on a 'face' for the audience. Be natural and relaxed. Use your face to give the audience feedback. Encourage participation with a friendly look, and provide positive reinforcement with a smile.

Gestures

Gestures improve communication (Graham and Argyle 1975; Riseborough 1981), and aid the comprehension of explanations and descriptions (Rogers 1978). They are also useful to focus the attention of the audience on the presenter. Research has shown that appropriate use of gesture helps memory and lends the speaker more credibility (Woodall and Burgoon 1981). The presenter who uses gesture effectively is likely to be perceived as interesting and enthusiastic.

Here are some examples of how gestures might be used:

- To replace certain words or phrases. (The shrug of the shoulders with hands held out, palms up, means 'I don't know'.)
- To give emphasis to key features of an explanation. (A firm chopping movement of the hands add emphasis to key words.)

- ◦ To direct the attention of the audience. (Pointing out items of interest on a diagram.)
- ◦ To illustrate objects or events. (Fist smashing into the palm of the other hand to indicate a crash.)
- ◦ To show the size or shape of an object. (The hands can indicate a circular shape. The width between the hands show different lengths.)
- ◦ To show a movement. (An undulating movement of the hands represents waves on the sea.)
- ◦ To demonstrate spatial relationships. (One hand under the other indicates 'underneath'.)
- ◦ To show an action. (There are many examples of gestures used to represent actions including smoking, drinking, and driving.)
- ◦ To indicate numbers. (Using the digits to indicate the first, second and third point of your explanation.)
- ◦ To represent an abstract idea or thought. (Using the two hands to weigh up alternative ideas.)

Remember you may use gestures unconsciously that give away information about how you are feeling. Adjusting the knot of your tie or playing with your ring may signal anxiety. Give your hands something to do. Hold a pen, or rest one hand on the lectern.

When using gestures:

- ◦ Be natural
- ◦ Avoid repetitive mannerisms
- ◦ Feel comfortable.

Do not use gestures just for the sake of it. Movements of the hands and arms that lack any purpose will only distract the audience.

Posture

Posture reflects the self-esteem of the individual. Slouched shoulders with the head down suggests boredom or a lack of confidence. Head up with shoulders back gives the impression of confidence.

A posture that is too static or too rigid is as uninviting as fidgeting and constant pacing. To find a balanced position try this exercise.

Stand with your legs apart with your feet pointing ahead and in line with your hips. Keep your head in the mid line and your shoulders down and relaxed. Gently rock forward until you feel as if you are going to lose your balance. Return to your central position. Repeat this movement to each side and backwards.

This should have given you a feel for your natural centre of balance. Even slight movements away from this central point create tension as the body tries to maintain its balance.

Positioning and orientation

This is about where you stand, and in what direction you face. This may sound a silly statement. Surely you stand in front of the audience? Most of the time you will do this, unless you are operating a slide projector from the back of the room. Slide projectors and other audio-visual aids are the Achilles heel for the presenter. You can probably think of many examples of poor positioning by speakers when using an audio-visual aid. The teacher who talks to the board as he writes. The presenter who turns to read each overhead. The lecturer who mutters into her demonstration model. Always face your audience when you are operating your aids. If necessary, memorise your slides and overheads to avoid having to turn and look at them. Face the audience when pointing to items on a white-board or flip chart. Avoid obstructing the audience's view of the board. Try these tips:

If you are right-handed:

Stand with the board or chart on your left side using your left hand to point out items

Start writing or drawing about a third of the way in so you cover less as you draw or write.

If you are left-handed:

Stand with the board or chart on your right side using your right hand to point out items

Write or draw on the first two-thirds of the board, leaving the last third (the part nearest you) clear.

(Watch the weather reporters on television to see how a professional does it!)

Positioning is important. It is tempting to hide behind the lectern or the overhead projector if you are nervous. However, this is exactly the message it signals to the audience. Be bold. Step out and claim your spot. Do not let your equipment become a barrier between you and the audience, either physically or psychologically.

Annoying habits

Everyone has an idiosyncratic gesture, expression or tone of voice. These are the characteristics that make up our individual identities. Some of these behaviours only occur at times of stress or anxiety.

During a presentation these habits can sometimes become exaggerated, and on occasions intensely irritating to the audience. One predictor of whether your habits will offend is the frequency with which they occur. A friend or colleague can help point out your more annoying mannerisms. Otherwise viewing yourself on video tape will provide immediate enlightenment. These are some annoying habits noticed by the author in various presenters:

- Scratching, rubbing or picking at various body parts!
- Tapping a pen in the cleft of their chin
- Pushing up rolled sleeves
- Teeth sucking
- Vocal mannerisms
- Pacing
- Jangling keys in the pocket.

Other common habits to watch out for include:

- Excessive grooming of hair
- Pushing at the knot of your tie
- Lack of eye-contact
- Flicking hair back off the face
- Continuously checking their watch for the time
- Umming and aaing
- Nervous cough or laugh.

Action Points

(1) Think about the presentations and lectures that you have attended. Did the presenters have any annoying habits? Why did it make you feel this way?

(2) Watch politicians giving speeches. Do their gestures match their words? Are there any gestures you associate with a particular person?

(3) Think about your own non-verbal behaviour. If someone were to mimic you, what characteristic traits would they be able to exaggerate? These might be gestures, posture or facial expression.

(4) Watch speakers on the television, at lectures or conferences. Make a conscious note of how and when they use gestures. Study your presentation. Are there any places where you can make use of gesture?

(5) Ask a friend to watch the rehearsal of your presentation. Ask her to check your eye-contact, facial expression and use of gestures.

Summary Points

- Use eye-contact to establish rapport with the audience, and demonstrate your interest and sincerity.

- Look at the audience for feedback on their level of understanding, interest and motivation.

- Avoid giving mixed messages. Match your facial expression to your verbal message.

- Gestures improve communication by clarifying and illustrating explanations and descriptions.

- Posture reflects self-esteem. Aim to develop a natural, balanced posture.

- ○ Face the audience when talking. Do not hide behind your audio-visual aids.

- ○ Identify your annoying mannerisms and try to eradicate them from your performance.

21

Effective use of Audio-Visual Materials

There will be many factors influencing your choice of audio-visual aid including cost, ease of use, availability, the nature of your presentation and personal preference. This section will help you to choose the appropriate audio-visual aids for your presentation and show you how to use them more effectively.

What is available?

A wide range of audio-visual aids are available. These include:

- Whiteboard
- Flip chart
- Overhead projector
- Slide projector
- Video playback
- Audio playback
- Multi-media
- Realia (real objects)
- Models.

Whiteboard

A whiteboard, or dry write board, is a common feature in most training facilities. It functions as a useful notepad for recording spontaneous comments or for drawing pictures and diagrams to illustrate a point. (Special non-permanent markers are required.) It can also be used as a noticeboard, for example, listing general reference material for the audience. Drawbacks include the need to erase material before new information can be added, and the difficulty in preparing material in advance. They are relatively low cost items.

Flip chart

A flip chart consists of a large notepad fixed to a stand. It is a cheap and familiar training aid, which is often used as a notepad for workshop or seminar discussions. Large flip charts are difficult to transport but smaller, desktop varieties are available. These are handy for preparing material in advance, but their small size restricts their use to groups of ten or less. The flip chart has an advantage over the white board in that information can be retained for future reference.

Overhead projector

An overhead projector (OHP) is probably the most flexible and widely used of all the audio-visual aids. It projects written or printed images from acetate sheets onto a screen in an enlarged form. Acetates are easy to prepare and are particularly useful for displaying pie charts, graphs and other illustrations. Its operation is relatively simple, although projection screens can present difficulties! There is a limit to the amount of information that can be portrayed at any one time, and it is less suitable for large auditoriums. Machines that have an acetate roll attached can be used as a notepad by the presenter. This has the advantage of allowing the presenter to face the audience whilst making notes. Portable models are available.

Slide projector

A slide projector, like the OHP, projects images onto a screen. Slides are the source of the image rather than an acetate. The colour of text and background on slides varies, each one having advantages and disadvantages.

Black text on a white background is easy to read, but can cause eye-strain. It is visible with fairly light conditions.

White text on a black background needs very dark conditions to be readable.

(If you have access to a computer you can see the effect of changing the background colour. Most computers have black text on a white background. Select a section of text by highlighting it, which will create white text on a black background. Compare reading it with the room light on, and then off.)

Blue text on a white background is easier on the eye, but needs a moderately dark room to be visible. Blue-on-white is probably the best choice if you have a large number of slides to show.

A slide projector is preferable to an OHP for large auditoriums and audiences, and some material, for example histology, may be better represented as slides. As slides need to be prepared in advance there is limited scope for altering the display apart from omitting or changing the order of presentation. Lighting needs to be dimmed and this can make note taking difficult for the audience and prevent you from seeing your notes.

Anyone who has attended a presentation involving the use of a slide projector will know that there are a number of pitfalls. Smooth operation takes practice. The logistics of operating the projector can create a barrier between the speaker and the audience, and it is therefore less appropriate for informal talks where interaction is desirable.

Video playback

Video playback requires a video player and a television or monitor. Large audiences or detailed visual images require a large sized screen. This is a point not always appreciated by organisers. Check the dimensions of the equipment, the potential size of the audience and the acoustics before using any video material. Larger images can be produced using a video projector and screen. The screens can also be positioned higher up and are therefore more visible to people at the back of the audience. However, a projector needs a darker room, which can make note taking difficult. Always check the compatibility of your video tape with the available equipment. If you are planning to record your own film material, speak to your media resources department first.

Audio playback

Audio playback equipment is available in various forms that include cassette recorders, reel to reel, digital audio tape (DAT) player, and public address systems. You may be tempted to use your personal machine, especially if it is portable. However, it is unlikely that this has either adequate volume or quality for a sizeable audience. Check what is available at the venue. Public address systems are the best option or ask for a playback system that has speakers. It is always difficult to produce good quality recordings as an amateur. Sophisticated equipment with expensive microphones is required to achieve a professional recording level. However, the more sophisticated the equipment the more things can go wrong during recording. Seek advice from your media resources department before attempting to make recordings for public presentations.

Table 4.1 Table for common audio-visual aids and their specific features

audio-visual aid	power source	portable models	technical support	lighting needs to be dimmed	audience size		
					10	10–50	>50
OHP	•	•	•		•	•	
Full size flip chart		•			•	•	
Desk top flip chart		•			•		
Whiteboard					•	•	
Slide projector	•		•	•	•	•	•
Audio playback	•	•	•		•	•	•
Video playback	•		•	•	•	•	•*
Realia/ models		•			•		
Multi-media	•		•	•	•	•+	

+ with LCD screen   * with projector screen

Realia and models

Realia (real objects) or models can greatly enhance a presentation and encourage audience interaction. A wide range of excellent anatomical models are now available. Demonstration of procedures, treatment and therapy may be more appropriately explained using the actual equipment. Keep demonstration copies of equipment to ensure that they are readily available. This helps to make sure that the parts are kept together in an orderly fashion. Objects and models work best with smaller audiences of ten or less.

Multi-media packages

These are computer based packages and consist of a combination of text, graphics, video and audio information shown in real time. This is a fast growing area that allows the computer user to interact and control what is happening on the screen. For example, text can be added or deleted and animated sequences created. It is most effective as an interactive tool and therefore it is more suited to small groups of ten or less. If you need to use it with larger audiences, a liquid crystal display projection panel is necessary. This fits onto the stage of an OHP and projects the image onto a large screen. However this does limit the complexity of material that can be shown. Presenters can use this equipment to prepare material for training packages to be used independently by students.

Choosing audio-visual aids for your presentation

Use the Table 4.1 to help you select your audio-visual equipment:

Preparing material for audio-visual aids

How much text?

One of the most common mistakes made by presenters is to have over-crowded visuals. These are difficult to read from the back of the room, and leave the audience no time to assimilate information from either the acetate or the speaker. Between six to ten lines of text is the recommended maximum for acetates and slides. Keep text central to the acetate or slide, as the lower edge of acetates is often obstructed.

What size of text?

Visuals are meant to be seen and read, even from the back of the room. Therefore letters, and the spaces between lines need to be large. Below is an example of minimum text size (font size 24) for an acetate:

about this size

Remember the size of your audience dictates the size of your text.

What style of text is best?

Some fonts or letter styles are more suitable for use on visuals. Simple plain lettering is usually more successful. Choose a style that has fairly broad strokes. It needs to be of medium density or in bold.

Use a mixture of upper and lower case. Only use uppercase for labelling graphics or where there is a mixture of letters and numerals.

Use a change in style to highlight key points or to add visual interest. However, avoid the temptation to create fancy displays using a variety of fonts. These may look attractive but make the text difficult to read. Two styles are sufficient for each visual. For example, the titles in one style and the rest of the text in another. The golden rule is 'Be consistent'.

Why would I want to use colour?

Colour can add interest and help the audience understand information faster. It can help structure your visual aid and guide the audience's attention. Use it to:

- Add visual interest
- Distinguish between items
- Colour code items that are the same or are related to each other
- Highlight key words in the text
- To help the audience identify which points are primary and which are secondary
- Identify headings and sub-headings
- Indicate the significance of an item.

How do I choose colours?

In everyday life the choice of colours is often dictated to us by tradition and culture. When an English couple marries it is traditional that the bride wears white, and at a funeral English people are expected to dress in black. Individuals also make choices. These personal preferences are linked to the physical properties of different colours, and the images and emotions connected with them. Some colours are brighter and 'stand out', providing sharp contrasts. Others are more subtle and blend in with the background. Colours can also be perceived differently depending on the colour next to them.

The images and emotions that colours evoke differ widely between individuals. To one person red may symbolise a political party, another may think of bloodshed, whilst a third may associate it with sex.

Different cultures will use colour in different ways, so that in some Asian countries red clothing is worn at marriages, and in China white is worn at funerals. A colour combination may have a strong association with certain objects. In a hospital yellow and black are associated with radioactivity. Choosing colours for impact, to promote an idea or sell a product can be challenging unless you know your audience well.

Despite this, there are some rules which are familiar to any home decorator, about the use of colour. These rules can be illustrated by the colour wheel. This is an idea originally developed by Isaac Newton. The wheel is based on the three pure colours of red, blue and yellow. These are also known as the primary colours. The rest of the wheel is made up of secondary and tertiary colours. A secondary colour is made by mixing equal amounts of two primaries. Red and yellow make orange, blue and yellow make green, and blue and red make violet. The tertiary colours are made up of equal amounts of primary and secondary colours. For example, yellow added to green makes lime green. There are twelve colours in total. All other colours are derived from either mixing together the basic colours of the wheel, or adding black or white to them. You can find colour wheels in most decorating books.

Use the following information to help guide you when choosing colours for your visuals:

- Dark colours (black, dark green, dark blue) and warm colours (red, orange) advance or stand out

- Cool colours recede or fade into the background (for example, pale blue, aqua and pale green)

- Colours opposite each other on the colour wheel contrast most strongly (for example, red with green, yellow with blue)

- Harmonious colours lie close to each other on the colour wheel (for example blue, blue green and aqua)

- Subtle colours are a mixture of two or more pure colours (for example, orange with some blue)

○ Changing the lightness or darkness of colours creates different tones, e.g. pink, red and maroon.

How do I use colour on visuals?

○ Use primary or contrasting colours to differentiate between two items. For example, lines on a graph.

○ Use harmonious colours to differentiate between several items. For example, on a bar chart or pie chart.

○ Use dark or warm colours to highlight. For example, key words on a text slide.

○ Use bright or warm colours to accentuate. For example, to make a small drawing stand out.

○ Use subtle colours for large items or areas. For example, large drawings or as a background colour.

○ Use cool colours on words or numerals that have less importance. For example, less important figures in a table.

Remember:

○ Use a maximum of four colours on a visual.

○ Avoid red and green together because of colour blindness.

○ Be consistent. Use the same colours for items throughout your visuals, e.g. green for population figures, drugs in red.

○ Avoid camouflaging effects, e.g. using two colours of the same tone, e.g. pink on a red background.

○ Colour used on a black background requires very dark conditions.

○ Yellow on white is difficult to see.

How can I display numerical information?

Numerical information is much more digestible for an audience when it is presented in a pictorial way such as a pie chart or bar graph. This way any patterns can easily be identified and comparisons between data is quick and easy.

Keep the amount of information displayed to a minimum by only selecting relevant data, and using several visuals if necessary. It is better to display several simple charts than confuse the audience with an 'impressive' but over complex chart. It is important to choose a visual display that suits your numerical data and your purpose. See *Presenting Your Research* for ideas on displaying numerical data.

I would like to include some drawings

Drawings are useful to show objects that are difficult to visualise or to add humour in the form of a cartoon. Objects that are too large for display can be drawn instead, and the detail of a small item enlarged in an illustration.

Drawings might be:

- A cartoon
- An outline
- To scale, such as a building plan
- Schematic, such as an organisational chart or diagram
- Figurative; this is where a symbol represents an idea or an object
- Representative – the main features of an object are portrayed.

Drawings and illustrations in books are often too small and complex to be reproduced successfully on an acetate or slide. Software programmes are available that can help you generate images. A simpler method is tracing paper and pencil.

Keep drawings simple with bold lines. Colour can be used to help define the image or emphasise important parts. Small objects need brighter colours while larger items are better in more subtle colours. Try out various combinations and view them at a distance. This will help you make the right choice.

How can I make my visuals more attractive?

You can add interest by varying the format, so that the text is not all in paragraphs or a series of numbered points. Another way of adding interest is to use colour. (See the section above about using colour.)

Note that it is sometimes difficult to predict exactly how people will perceive your visuals. What seems perfectly clear to you, creates confusion and annoyance in the audience. Using a bold line on a graph might falsely suggest it has more importance than the other dotted or thinner lines. A star or tick in a table may be taken to indicate approval where none is intended. Careful preparation will help guard against these sorts of errors. Showing your material to other people is invaluable, as it often elicits information about ambiguous phrasing and images.

How can I print my acetates?

Printed acetates instantly add an air of professionalism, and indicate to the audience that considerable thought and preparation have been involved. You will find that ordinary typescript is too small to be read at a distance, so avoid photocopying straight from printed material or using ordinary type-written script.

Acetates can be prepared by using a computer that has the facility to enlarge text and add appropriate styles and formats. Software programmes are available that can formulate graphs, pie charts and tables. Check the facilities on both your computer and your printer.

You can either print your work on plain paper and photocopy this onto an acetate sheet, or print directly onto the acetate sheet itself. First check that your photocopier or printer can cope with acetates. You will also need acetates specifically designed for this purpose.

How can I make my audio tapes sound professional?

It is worth spending some time preparing good quality demo tapes as you will be able to use them repeatedly, thus saving on preparation time in the future. One of the main difficulties with amateur tapes is the amount of background noise. Often footsteps and voices in the corridor outside the recording room are exaggerated on the tape. Try to find a quiet room that has absorbent surfaces, such as carpets, soft furnishings and carpets. Position the tape recorder on a separate table.

Use a plug-in microphone as this delivers a much better quality of recording than built in microphones. There is some disagreement about the best type of microphone. A lapel microphone enables the distance between the microphone and speaker's voice to remain constant. However, there can be problems with clothes rub. This is the noise of clothing moving over the microphone. Hand held models can intimidate the subject of your recording and recording levels may be varied if the microphone is moved around. A good compromise is to have a microphone on a stand placed between the people being recorded.

Always have a rehearsal before you start the actual recording, so you can check whether your machine is picking up any extraneous noises. If you have built up several tapes that you need to play at one presentation, try to edit your material onto one tape. This will save you from carrying around lots of different tapes and ensures a smoother transition from one example to another. Once you have made your recording, break the tab at the back of the tape to ensure against accidental erasure.

What do I need to remember about preparing video tapes?

Make sure you have the written permission of the participants, and that it has been made clear that it is intended for use in a presentation. Aim for the best quality recording. There are three points that affect quality (1) the video tape; (2) the camcorder; (3) playback facility – video recorder and the television monitor. A good recording can sound disastrous on a poor quality video recorder, and a high quality television screen will not mask a poor quality recording.

As with audio tapes, the use of an external mike is recommended. Tripods help to stabilise the camcorder and although they reduce flexibility, are preferable to trying to hold the camera. Leave a blank stretch of tape lasting for several seconds between recordings. This will allow time to put the tape on stop or pause without affecting the running of your piece.

Hints for using audio-visual aids

These guidelines give hints on how to present effectively with your chosen audio-visual aids. You should also consult with your media representatives either at work or at the venue of your proposed presentation. They can offer you specific advice and assist you on the day. Tell the organiser about your audio-visual requirements well before the presentation.

General Hints

- **Safety Hint** – Remember to check for trailing leads from OHP, video and other electrical equipment. Position equipment with leads out of the way or taped to the floor if you are installing equipment as a permanent feature. (In the latter case, take care to position the equipment correctly in the first place.)

- Check power points. Are there enough? Where are they? Do not overload power points.

- Check lighting and light switches. Is there a dimmer switch? Which switches operate which lights?

- Portable projection screens (like deck chairs) are not always easy to assemble so find out *how* before your talk.

- Check equipment is working. Is the plug in? Are all the switches on?

Whiteboard

- Check that your writing is legible from the back of the room, and that all the participants have a clear view of the board.

- Erase material with a damp cloth or sponge when you have finished, otherwise it may distract the audience.

- Remember to use the correct (non-permanent) marker pens. (If you use the wrong pen you will need a cleaning agent to remove the marks.) Bring your own spare pens.

- Remember that you can attach material to metal backed boards using magnets.

Flip chart

- Position the flip chart before you start talking.

- Check your writing is legible from the back of the room, and that all the participants have a clear view of the chart.

- Keep a supply of coloured marker pens.

- Cover any material when you have finished otherwise it may distract the audience. Either mask with paper or leave blank pages in between the prepared sheets.

- Check there are enough clean sheets for your requirements.

- Fold back sheets rather than tearing them off, as you may need to refer to them.

Slide Projector

- Rehearse using the type of projector available for your presentation. Practise inserting and removing both the slides and the slide carousel.

- Number your slides in the sequence of presentation. It is also useful to make some marks that indicate which way up and which way round they should be loaded into the carousel.

- Use remote control so you are in front of the audience rather than behind.

- Avoid obstructing the audience's view of the screen, or standing between the projector and the screen.

- Remember slides are best seen in a darkened room, which may make it difficult for you to see your notes. There may be a light on the lectern, otherwise a small torch is a handy alternative.

- If a number of people are involved in the presentation, elect one member to be your assistant projectionist. This will free you from the mechanics to concentrate on delivering the content of the slides. Jay (1993) suggests the following guidelines for working with an assistant projectionist:

  - Assistant checks the slides against the presenter's script or notes

  - Slides are loaded into the carousel

  - Assistant re-checks slides against script or notes

  - No changes or cuts after final rehearsal

  - Have a 'breakdown procedure', for example if a slide sticks – Is it omitted or shown later?

Overhead projector

- Position your OHP before the start of your talk. Check the projected image is in focus and is visible from the back of the room. In some locations it may be necessary to dim the lighting.

- If you have shaky hands, use a pen to indicate items by laying it on the acetate rather than pointing. More extrovert presenters should be wary of pointers that wander, or wave like the conductor's baton!

- Points can be highlighted or added by writing on a clear acetate placed over your original. This technique can be used to build up a complex overhead from two or three simple ones. Alternatively you can slide your acetate under the roll of acetate on the machine and write on this.

- Let the audience see the whole of the acetate at least once, and then use a piece of paper to mask out material until it is needed. This helps to focus the audience's attention and controls the pace of the presentation.

- Do not try to compete with the noise of the OHP motor when making an important point. Switch it off. The audience will appreciate a rest from the noise as well.

- Devise a system for ordering your acetates. Always know where you put your last acetate, and where to get the next one. Filing acetates in a ring binder is one of the most effective ways of keeping them tidy. You will need a desk or chair near the OHP for your notes and acetates.

○ Acetates with a frame are less likely to curl up or float off the OHP. Use the frame for reminder notes.

○ Use the acetate roll as a notepad to record contributions from the audience. Find out which way the roll of acetate should be wound, so you can quickly find the clean part of the roll. (Check that there is still some clear acetate left.) Note that certain portable models do not have this facility.

○ Switch off the OHP when you have finished showing your acetates. Never leave a blank screen.

Video playback

○ Use the remote controls to avoid turning your back on the audience.

○ Put the tape on pause when commenting on a particular clip.

○ Space your video material out during the presentation to achieve the greatest impact.

○ Always try to use video recordings that have good sound and visual quality.

○ Viewing is improved if the lighting is dimmed, but may make note taking difficult for the audience.

○ Set sound levels on the television before the presentation.

○ Use the largest monitor screen available. A video projector that projects the image onto a screen may be better for larger audiences.

○ Keep your video tapes in order by numbering them in the sequence you wish to show them, or prepare a demonstration tape with selected clips edited ready for viewing.

○ Mark each tape box clearly with details of the video tape contents.

○ Explain to the audience what they will be watching and why.

Audio playback

○ Keep your audio tapes in order by numbering them in the sequence you wish to play them, or prepare a demonstration tape with selected clips edited ready to play.

- Mark each tape box clearly with details of the audio tape contents.
- Explain to the audience what they will be hearing and why.
- Space your audio material out during the presentation to achieve the greatest effect.
- Always try to use good quality audio recordings.
- Set sound levels before the presentation. The acoustics of a room will be affected by its size, shape, the number of people in the audience and the amount of absorbent surfaces, e.g. soft furnishings, carpets.
- Put the tape on pause when commenting on a particular clip.

Realia, models and equipment

- Inspect for breakages and missing parts before the presentation.
- Familiarise yourself with all the components and practise the demonstration on friends and family.
- Make sure you have enough objects to hand round if you plan to let the audience examine items.
- Allow time for the audience to examine the items before you move on to another point.
- Check you have the necessary requirements, e.g. power supply.

Multi-media

- Use a personal computer with a small group. Larger groups will need a liquid crystal display projection panel with OHP along with the computer.
- Check you have all the necessary electrical requirements, e.g. power sockets, adapter leads.
- Rehearse the procedures carefully.
- Be ready to improvise if there is a power cut or other equipment failure.
- Do not allow the equipment to take over the show. Remember to keep the purpose of your presentation in mind.

Checklist of audio-visual aids

Equipment required:

- ☐ Whiteboard
- ☐ Flip chart
- ☐ OHP
- ☐ Slide projector
- ☐ Audio playback
- ☐ Video playback
- ☐ LCD projection panel

Organiser informed of requirements ☐

List of Equipment for Presentation:

Markers

- ☐ OHP pens (non-permanent in assorted colours)
- ☐ Whiteboard markers (assorted colours)
- ☐ Board eraser
- ☐ Large felt-tip pens

Visual Aids

- ☐ Prepared acetates
- ☐ Spare acetates
- ☐ Audio Tapes
- ☐ Video Tapes
- ☐ Slides
- ☐ Charts
- ☐ Anatomical Models
- ☐ ....
- ☐ ....
- ☐ ....

☐ Test or Assessment Materials

☐ ....

☐ ....

☐ ....

☐ Treatment or therapy equipment

☐ ....

☐ ....

☐ ....

Other items:

☐ Pointer

☐ Hand-outs

☐ Spare Paper

Name of Media Resources Officer/Equipment Technician:..
Tel No:..

Summary Points

○ There will be many factors influencing your choice of audio-visual aid including cost, ease of use, availability, the nature of your presentation and personal preference.

○ A wide range of audio-visual aids are available. These include whiteboard, flip chart, overhead projector, slide projector, video playback, audio playback, multi-media, realia (real objects) and models.

○ Visuals are 'visuals'. Choose the most legible size, font and style of text. Keep them simple.

○ Use colour to add interest and help the audience understand information faster.

- ◦ Choose colours on the basis of their natural properties. For example, highlight text by using a warm colour, which will stand out.
- ◦ Display numerical information with graphs or pie charts. Keep the amount of information displayed to a minimum by only selecting the relevant data.
- ◦ Aim for the highest quality for all of your technical equipment.
- ◦ Rehearse your procedures thoroughly. Practise using equipment.
- ◦ Order your materials into the sequence you will be using them, and mark all files, tape boxes clearly with the contents.
- ◦ Be aware of safety factors.
- ◦ Locate all the power points and light switches at the venue and check equipment is working before your presentation.
- ◦ Check your audio-visual aids are visible and audible at the back of the room.
- ◦ Bring any spare pens, acetates and so on with you.

Presentation Skills in Context
Client/Carer Workshops

As health professionals we are involved in developing and extending the knowledge and skills of our clients. We want them to understand their health problems and be actively involved in their treatment. Advice and information may be given directly to the client at clinic appointments, during a hospital stay or on a home visit. This may involve family or carers in some instances. In addition to this, workshops are increasingly being offered to both clients and carers. These focus on preventative work, rehabilitation, and health promotion. This chapter focuses on presenting or leading such a workshop.

The workshop can be based on real life experiences shared by the participants or on material prepared by the leader. Workshops usually involve lots of group activities thus providing the opportunity for:

- Experiences to be shared
- Knowledge to be shared
- Attention to shift away from the individual to the group
- Generating ideas
- Fostering a group identity
- The individual to gain support from others
- Discovering the different perspectives on a problem or on the solution of that problem
- Networking
- Individuals to take an active role in their health care.

Accommodation
The type and size of accommodation will have a significant impact on the success of your workshop. There needs to be adequate space for the whole

group plus additional spaces for small group activities. At least one large room is required. This should be big enough to allow the group to spread out and work in pairs or small groups, but not so large it seems inhospitable. You will also need several additional spaces that provide an opportunity for participants to work away from a large group.

Many training centres have the ideal set-up for workshops, and it is well worth spending some extra money to book these facilities. If you have to use other accommodation, try to ensure the rooms you are using are situated reasonably close together. This will save you time when you are supervising activities. Sound proofing is very important. Participants may not want to be overheard, nor do they want to be restrained from making a noise for fear of disturbing others.

Seating

Some consideration needs to be given to the type of chairs you use, as participants will be seated for much of the time. Your choice of seating will depend on the nature of your workshop. Soft armchairs are best for support groups. Other types of workshops require more upright chairs. It helps the organisation of activities if they are also easy to move around. Whatever your choice of chairs they need to be comfortable.

Make sure you have enough chairs, including some spares. This may seem a simple point but is easily overlooked. Some activities may require participants to work at tables. Again check there are enough to accommodate the whole group.

Think about the lay-out of seating. At the beginning of the session place the chairs in a circle or semi-circle. This format is more likely to increase interaction. A semi-circle is better if you are using audio-visual aids, as everybody will be facing the right way. At other times a circle can be used.

Using audio-visual aids

Organise your audio-visual requirements well in advance. Useful items for practical exercises include large sheets of paper (poster size), several large felt tips in assorted colours, Blu-Tac, pens and paper.

Choose audio-visual aids that maximise interaction between participants, and between participants and the workshop leader. Some of the most useful aids are flip charts, overhead projectors and whiteboards. For activities involving role plays, a camcorder and video playback facility are invaluable.

Arrive early on the day to arrange seating and set up your equipment. It may be sensible to bring a spare of any piece of equipment that is vital. If you are bringing your own audio-visual aids, check these are working at least two weeks before the event. Repair work or ordering parts takes time.

Planning the programme

The basic format for a workshop might look something like this.

A Workshop to Teach Life Saving Skills

- Introduction
- A statement about the importance of learning resuscitation skills
- Outline of the skills to be covered
- Demonstration and practical experience
- Summary
- Recommendations for applying skill in real life situations

You need to have a plan of what you are going to do and how long it will take. Otherwise it is easy for the workshop to become top heavy and activities at the start get large chunks of time, whilst activities near the end are rushed and too brief. Work out the duration of each activity including time to set it up and the feedback session. Remember that if it takes one individual three minutes to give feedback this is multiplied to thirty minutes with a group of ten.

Think about what point in the programme is best for each activity. Plan something lively for periods when the group's concentration will be flagging, such as after lunch or at the end of the day. Wait until the group have had an opportunity to gel together before introducing activities that involve personal disclosures.

The following example illustrates how the nature of an activity will influence when you use it with the group. These are two activities aimed at helping people to find out something about each other.

(1) Talk with your partner for five minutes and find out three things about them.

(2) Draw a picture of how you are feeling at the moment. When you have finished, share your pictures with each other as a group. Explain why you have drawn the different images.

The first activity is a superficial and light-hearted introduction. The second is a much more in-depth disclosure for the individual. This is partly because it is about feelings, but also the nature of the task. Drawing is a powerful tool. It is difficult to get away with just saying 'I'm fine'. The first activity is useful as a warm-up game. The second needs to be introduced once the group are more comfortable with working together.

Time-table breaks for refreshments and lunch. Include half-an-hour at the start of the workshop for people to have coffee and a chat. (This also helps you to deal with late comers, so that everyone is there at the start of the actual programme.)

Give participants a less detailed version of your plan as an agenda. This should state the start and finish times for each session. Remember to include your half hour session on the programme. This can be described as follows:

9.00-9.30. Registration (Coffee and Biscuits available)

Workshop manual

Prepare a workshop manual. This can be as simple as an A4 ring folder filled with all the material relevant to your course. This is particularly useful when you are working with someone else, as it can be quickly referred to for information. The following items are useful to include:

- Outline of the programme
- Aims and objectives for the workshop
- Copy of workshop leader's aide-memoire for the presentation
- Notes on each activity for the workshop leader(s)that include:
  - Title of the activity
  - The aims of the activity
  - Materials required
  - Length of the activity
  - Description of how to carry out the activity
  - Instructions to be given to the participants.
- Notes on each activity for the participants that include:
  - Title of the activity
  - The aims of the activity
  - Length of the activity

- Instructions for the activities.
- Copies of overheads, handouts, etc.
- Copy of the course evaluation form
- Checklist of audio-visual aids
- List of participants.

Organising activities

Here are a few tips on how to organise activities so that they run smoothly.

- The ideal number of participants for a workshop is between twelve to fifteen people. Plan activities around these numbers, and make contingency plans if fewer people attend than expected.

- Help people to get to know each other by providing sticky name labels. People can write their names on the labels as they arrive for the workshop.

- Start by setting some ground rules. These will depend on the nature of your activities. For example, where people are disclosing personal details, the group may decide to have a rule about confidentiality. Use a brainstorm (see below) to elicit ideas. The group are more likely to adhere to rules they have suggested than to ones imposed by the group leader.

- During games or set activities avoid assigning roles to particular individuals (Bond 1986). Ask people to divide into small groups first. Then they can decide amongst themselves who will be A, B, or C, and so on. The leader can then assign the roles to the letters, for example, the observer is A, the mother is B and the child is C.

- There are a number of different ways of choosing people for small group activities. A simple way is to go round the group and give each person in turn one of three numbers. For example 1, 2, or 3. All the people with number 1 are in group one, and so on. You may want to allocate people according to other factors, so that groups have a mixture of people. If so, provide lists of names and groups.

- Prepare signs to indicate in which rooms or spaces you are expecting small group activities to take place. This can just be a letter on a sheet of paper, for example group (1) placed on the appropriate door.

- Give the group instructions at the beginning of the activity. If it is small group work, wait until people have been assigned to their groups. Photocopy instructions for activities and hand these out to participants for reference.

Workshop activities

Here are some suggestions for activities that are useful for the workshop format:

Whole group activities

(1) Warm-up activities

- **'What's My Name?'** – The group form a circle and throw a soft toy or ball to each other. They must name the catcher before they throw the ball. This is a good game to help people to get to know each other's name.

- **'Who Is Your Neighbour?'** – Each person has to find out three things about their neighbour. You can provide the group with ideas (such as name, occupation), or let them choose their own. In some workshops you might want the pairs to explore questions such as 'What do they want out of the workshop?' 'What anxieties do they have about the workshop?' Allow each person five minutes to find out the relevant information. At the end each person has two minutes to introduce their partner to the group.

- **'Spot the Coincidence'** – Each pair has to find out what they have in common. You could set a target of three or four coincidences. The timing and structure are the same as for the above activity.

Aim to make these activities as quick as possible. Ideally they should last for 5–10 minutes only. Set the tone for the workshop by sticking rigidly to your timing.

(2) Brainstorming

This activity elicits words or phrases from the group in response to a specific topic or idea. Each participant in the group is asked to make a contribution. This ensures that everyone is involved in the process and avoids domination by a few of the more extrovert members. The responses are recorded by the group leader on a whiteboard, an overhead projector or a flip chart. (Writing on an overhead projector has the advantage of allowing the presenter to remain facing the front whilst writing. The projected image is also much larger and therefore more easily read.) At this stage it is important to treat all contributions as valid, otherwise some participants may feel excluded or embarrassed. Record comments verbatim if possible. The activity works best when a fast pace is maintained. Avoid debating individual points during the brainstorm. The results can be used later as a basis for a discussion.

Brainstorming is a good initial activity for a workshop. It can be used as:

- A starting point for discussion, e.g. 'How might a person who is HIV positive be discriminated against?'

- A way of eliciting lots of ideas in a short amount of time, e.g. tips on how to stop smoking.

- To negotiate an agenda for the workshop.

- To help with problem solving, e.g. ideas on how to improve finding medical records.

(3) Demonstration

Practical skills or behaviours are most effectively taught by instruction. A demonstration can be recorded on video, or carried out in front of the audience by the workshop leader or a group member.

There are advantages and disadvantages to both methods. Pre-recorded material guarantees that the demonstration will 'work', and frees the leader to discuss particular aspects with the group. However, a live presentation usually offers the participants a better view of what is actually happening. The demonstrator can also respond to the needs of the group by repeating actions, or comparing the wrong way of doing something with the right way. This is particularly true of situations where the group are simultaneously attempting to copy the actions of the demonstrator.

Learning is enhanced if individuals have the opportunity to practise the skills under the guidance of the demonstrator. The ideal situation is for the group to be copying each step of the demonstration as it is happening. Unfortunately this is not always practicable.

Another method is for the workshop leader to repeat the demonstration with the group giving step by step instructions. Hand-outs containing written instructions for the demonstration can be provided for participants. These should be given out after the demonstration, otherwise participants will be reading and not watching the demonstration.

Planning a demonstration involves deciding what will be said and what will be done. Think about how you would explain tying shoe laces to someone, without the benefit of a demonstration or drawings. It would be a lengthy and very difficult explanation. Demonstrations are about actions. However, understanding is improved if these actions are also described in words; for example, 'Now, I am folding the bandage lengthways'. The group can also be alerted to the most salient aspects of the demonstration, for example 'Notice the type of knot I am using for this bandage'.

Any essential materials or equipment can be displayed at the beginning of the demonstration or introduced at appropriate times during the presentation. If you are unsure about making a demonstration then watch any cookery programme on television for some excellent examples of how it is done.

(4) Discussion

Discussion can be stimulated by asking specific questions or posing a problem, or it may arise from a brainstorming activity. This is an opportunity for people to share experiences, voice doubts or express opinions. Leading a discussion is not the exclusive role of the health professional, and may be carried out by a member of the group.

Potential problems may arise if one or two people dominate or the discussion lacks a focus. A good leader will ensure that individuals are drawn into the debate so that everyone is able to participate. Reminders can be given about time so the group are able to prioritise their discussion points. At the end the leader can help draw together ideas in a summary.

(5) Question and answer

This type of activity helps answer any specific queries participants might have. As information about a wide range of topics might be requested, it is difficult to prepare completely. One way of dealing with this is to ask for a list of questions earlier in the day. Although this may take away some of the spontaneity, it gives you time to prepare.

Use questions to check on what the group have understood. It will also help to uncover any myths or false beliefs, which can then be challenged.

(6) Problem solving

Problem solving is a practical way of addressing issues pertinent to the group members (Open University 1987). Ask the group to suggest difficulties or dilemmas they would like to problem solve. These need to be on going constant problems, rather than a one off incident. They also need to be issues that individuals are trying to deal with themselves. It should not be someone else's problem.

Select one individual's problem. Ask her to word the problem in a way that asks for a solution. So instead of 'My child is so naughty, he won't go to bed' use 'How can I get my child to go to sleep at bedtime?' Write this in the middle of a large flip chart or whiteboard.

Initially the group are allowed to ask specific questions to establish some of the background. For example, in the above problem they might ask what time the child went to bed or how many siblings did the child have. The group are not allowed to ask any 'Have you tried questions...'

Next, the group are asked to brainstorm solutions to the problem. At this stage the person who posed the problem does not respond in any way. All ideas are excepted and written round the outside of the question. This continues until the group have exhausted all their ideas.

The originator of the problem is then asked to look at the solutions. Any unsuitable ideas are crossed out. Stress to the group that the ideas might be OK, but are not appropriate for this individual. The remaining ideas are then placed in a hierarchy to indicate the order in which they will be tested. The person should be encouraged to talk about how she will implement the solutions.

(7) Modelling

Sometimes a 'good' model or role play is contrasted with a 'bad' model. Participants are encouraged to identify the skills or behaviours that differentiate the two. This can be very effective in showing people the difference between what they are doing and what they are aiming to do. Modelling is a very powerful tool, and professionals need to be cautious about setting unrealistic goals for participants.

Activities for small groups or pairs

(1) Brainstorming

An individual or two people working together can use this technique. The process is similar to the large group brainstorms with ideas or comments recorded quickly on a large sheet of paper. It is particularly useful for people who are nervous about sharing their ideas in a large group. The individual or paired brainstorm gives them some thinking time. Once the brainstorm is completed they can discuss it in a larger group.

(2) Posters

Small groups work on a particular theme or brainstorm. They are asked to prepare a poster, which is then displayed on the wall. In this way the group have the opportunity to consolidate their understanding, share ideas and learn from each other. It is also a way of checking on what members have gained from the workshop. Examples of poster activities include:

- ○ Designing a leaflet that advises on 'How to Live Life After a Bypass Operation'.
- ○ Brainstorming the emotions felt following a bereavement.
- ○ Drawing an advertisement for a technique for managing challenging behaviour. The group have to sell their idea to the rest of the group.

Role play and behavioural rehearsal

This technique is now a popular tool on many courses and workshops. It is also an activity that generates enormous anxiety in people. The workshop leader needs to bear this in mind and handle the activity sensitively. Role play is particularly useful for practising the skills required during day to day contact with other people. Examples are:

- ○ The parent learning to reinforce their child's good behaviour during a play session.
- ○ The disabled client who wants to learn to be more assertive with shop assistants.
- ○ The carer who is practising skills of giving advice to their clients.

It is useful to make a distinction between role play and behavioural rehearsal.

Behavioural rehearsal

This is the rehearsal or practise of a skill or a set of skills. These might be skills of asking questions, saying 'no' assertively, or expressing feelings to a loved one. The workshop leader or preferably the group members invent a scenario on which the role rehearsal is based. The idea is to provide a general context in which target skills can be developed. It is not based on a real life situation.

Role play

This is similar to behavioural rehearsal, in that a skill or set of skills are practised. The difference is that the scenario is based on a real event experienced by one of the participants. The context is very specific to the individual concerned, who guides other participants through the roles and dynamics encountered in the actual situation.

For example, a carer working with the elderly has had trouble in communicating with a client in his care. Although she is an intelligent lady she has difficulties in understanding speech following a recent stroke. Before her illness he had a close relationship with this lady. He is now finding conversation embarrassing and frustrating. He is attending the workshop to find out about strategies that help communication with speech impaired people. He wants to practise slowing down his speech and simplifying information. He is particularly anxious not to sound condescending.

The carer can first practise skills through behavioural rehearsal. In this way he has the opportunity to learn and develop skills without the added burden of his emotional reaction to the real life situation. The group members may want to contribute ideas for a scenario. This can be as far removed from the real life situation as a police officer giving instructions to a tourist who speaks very little English. The carer plays the police officer and a group member takes on the role of the tourist. The only restriction is that the scenario must elicit the target skills. In this case they are 'slowing down speech' and 'simplifying information'.

Once the carer is confident about using these skills he can try them out in a role play. Here one of the other members plays the client. The carer will give instructions on how to set up the role play. This will include information on the lay-out of furniture, the names of participants and a description of the client's communication. The carer is ready to role-play the real situation.

Getting into role

'Getting into role' is a concept that is very useful for role play situations. It is a bit like preparing for a role in a drama. It may seem a little silly at first, but it really helps to set the scene and get you into the mood. A more serious side is that it allows the role-players to dissociate any negative feelings from the real person. For example, they can express their anger towards the pretend person and not the group member.

To get into role each participant must describe who they are in terms of the role they are going to play. In the behavioural rehearsal described above, the member playing the tourist might say: 'I am a French student. I have brown hair and I am dressed casually in jeans and a tee-shirt.' In the role-play, the person role-playing the client might say: 'I am ninety years old with white hair. I tend to look confused when people speak to me.' The amount of detail will vary according to the needs of the different players.

Note I have used the word 'say'. It is important that the roles are said aloud to the group, as this is part of the process. You can help the process by asking people to 'go into role' or 'take the role'.

Once the role play is completed the players must come out of the role. This should be done before any discussion or attempt to provide feedback. Both participants must say 'I am coming out of role and returning to...' Here the participants should speak their name and any other details that seem appropriate.

The feedback stage

Part of the learning process in behavioural rehearsal and role play is receiving feedback. It is important that this feedback is provided in a systematic way. This involves several stages.

(1) The first stage is to increase the participants awareness of different behaviours or skills. The workshop leader can help by providing information, encouraging discussion and modelling behaviours.

(2) Simply knowing the behaviours is not sufficient. The participants need to be able to identify when it is appropriate to use these behaviours.

(3) Once the participants have an understanding of these behaviours, they need to try out these skills for themselves. Participants need to be active in selecting target behaviours for practice. These should not be imposed by the workshop leader.

(4) Behavioural rehearsal provides the opportunity for practice. It allows the participant to test out new skills, and observe the effects of their changed behaviour on others. This practice must be accompanied by feedback.

The group leader can help to elicit feedback. This should come first from the active member, and then from the recipient in the behavioural rehearsal. Finally the rest of the group can be invited to make comments and suggestions.

Feedback needs to be specific with an emphasis on reinforcing appropriate behaviours (Binstead 1986), rather than on highlighting any inadequacies in the participant's performance. Use the following strategies to help participants give effective feedback.

○ Prompt positive reinforcement – Ask what the participant did well. (Success can be measured by its effect on the recipient. Did the participant achieve her goal?)

○ Ask the group to be specific – So if someone comments 'He was assertive', ask for specific examples like 'he used a firm tone of voice' or 'he maintained eye-contact with the person'.

○ Increase the group's awareness of the target skills – Ask the group to choose certain behaviours or skills to observe during the rehearsal. They can record when and how often these behaviours occur, and the response of the recipient. For instance, observing when and how often verbal praise is used.

○ Encourage the participants to analyse the situation – How do they think the recipient is likely to react to certain behaviours? How did the recipient act?

○ Explore the participant's feelings – How did they feel? This includes the active member, the recipient and the rest of the group.

○ Ask for suggestions – It is a good rule to insist that if people have a comment to make, that they also offer a suggestion for change. For example, suggesting someone uses more facial expression to show that they are listening.

(5) Provide the opportunity for making comparisons – Allow the participant to repeat the experience. It is crucial that this happens within the same session. This helps the person to end on a note of success.

Summary Points

○ Workshops are an alternative method of providing support, information and training to clients and carers.

○ Group work has a number of advantages that include sharing of experiences and knowledge by the participants.

○ The type and size of accommodation will have a significant impact on the success of your workshop. There needs to be adequate space for large and small group activities. Seating needs to be arranged to maximise interaction.

○ Organise equipment needs well in advance. Flip charts, overhead projectors, camcorder and video playback are the most useful items.

- Plan the workshop to allow plenty of time for demonstrations and practical experience. Think carefully about when you time-table activities.

- Prepare a workshop manual. This will contain all the material and information relevant to your course.

- Activities for the workshop might be whole group activities such as a brainstorming session, or small group work such as preparing posters.

- Behavioural rehearsal is a form of role play that gives participants an opportunity to rehearse or practise a skill or a set of skills. The context used to practise the skills is based on a neutral real life experience.

- Role play uses scenarios that are based on a real event experienced by one of the participants. The context is very specific to the individual concerned.

- Feedback is an essential part of behavioural rehearsal and role play. It needs to be systematic and focused on specific skills.

Presentation Skills in Context
Presentations to Other Professionals

Many of your presentations will involve audiences who have a variety of professional backgrounds. Some of these may be health care disciplines; others may be from a variety of backgrounds such as social services and education. As a presenter you will have to meet the needs of these different groups. Part of the challenge is identifying what these needs are.

Here are five examples of presentations to different professional groups. Each one makes different demands on the presenter. What factors would you consider are important with these different audiences?

(1) A radiographer giving a lecture about her work to a group of student nurses.

(2) A speech therapist making a presentation entitled 'Communication Difficulties Following a Stroke' at a conference on rehabilitation. The audience is a mixture of medical and therapy disciplines.

(3) An occupational therapist presenting her research to a group of consultant paediatricians.

(4) A hearing therapist leading a workshop for social workers on 'Hearing Loss in the Elderly'.

(5) A clinical psychologist talking at a council meeting regarding the opening of a new community unit for disturbed adolescents. The audience includes local residents, the governor of the local school, the community police officer and representatives of the local shopkeepers' association.

The key factors are:

○ Knowledge base

○ Experience

- Skills
- Language (particularly terminology)
- Perspective
- Attitude
- Status.

Let's look at each example in turn.

Example 1

Although this lecture involves two different professional groups, this is a fairly straightforward presentation. The radiographer is talking to another group of health professionals, about a topic that is unlikely to be controversial. As the audience consists of students, the presenter will need to take into account their knowledge to date and their specific learning needs.

Example 2

This presentation involves not only speaking to other professionals, but professionals from several different disciplines. They will have a mixture of backgrounds, knowledge and experience. Although the audience and presenter have a mutual goal and shared interest in rehabilitation, each discipline will have a different perspective on the subject. They will all be experts in their field. The presenter will need to consider carefully the type of information and language that is accessible to all members of the audience.

Example 3

In this example the presenter is talking to a professional group who are often in a senior position to therapists. This may be daunting for some presenters. However, the audience are health professionals who will have a fairly good understanding of the occupational therapist's work. Dealing with nerves is probably the main factor.

Example 4

The professionals in this audience have a non-health background. The model for delivery of care is distinct from the health model. There are differences in approach, as well as language and terminology. The presenter needs to avoid unnecessary jargon, although some technical terms will have to be introduced for the audience to make sense of the subject matter. Preparation of the content will involve identifying the needs of the audience. The presenter will have to find answers to questions like 'What is their day-to-day contact with the elderly?', 'What difficulties do they come across with people who are hard of hearing?', 'What do they know about hearing loss already?'

Example 5

The content of this presentation is emotive. The presenter is likely to be greeted with a mixture of attitudes, some of which will be negative. They may include hostility, concern, and anxiety. A mixed audience will also have a range of concerns. The presenter will have to deal with each one. The presenter will need to anticipate likely objections and prepare responses. A significant part of the presentation will include time for questions. Providing examples of other successful community units would definitely be an advantage for this presenter.

There are some general points to take into consideration with any audience. These are:

Background knowledge, skills and experience

It is difficult to predict assumed knowledge when you are dealing with an audience from a mixture of backgrounds. There is the double fold danger of either pitching your presentation at either too high or too low a level. The presenter has to present material in a way that is understandable by everyone, but is not irritatingly patronising to the more knowledgeable individuals. Always acknowledge the expertise of these individuals.

Language

You will need to select your vocabulary carefully, so that the words you use do not confuse or offend the audience. Always avoid jargon.

Perspective

You need to identify what areas of your subject matter are of interest to the audience. Find out their expectations and attitudes. Why have you been asked? This will give you some ideas.

Mixed audiences will also have different perspectives on the same topic. For example, therapists attending a presentation on the management of swallowing difficulties following a stroke will have different needs and interests. Each one will have a different perspective on the client's difficulties, although they will all share the common goal of managing feeding and swallowing. The physiotherapist is involved in the management of posture, respiration and movement. The dietician is concerned with nutrition. The focus of the speech therapist is on rehabilitating the swallowing mechanism. There will also be areas where the roles of the professional cross over.

How can you prepare for your presentation?

Research your audience

It is essential to do your homework on finding out about your audience. Ask the organisers of the talk about what they hope the audience will gain from the talk. Try to find out some specific details about the participant's knowledge and experience.

Rehearse your presentation

Enlist the help of a friend or colleague who has a similar background or interests as your prospective audience. Ask them to listen to your presentation. This will give you some idea of how your audience will react to the content and delivery.

Ask them to use this checklist to help give you feedback:

- Are there any words or phrases that are unfamiliar?
- Are explanations clear? Do they need to be simpler? Do you need more examples?
- Will the content of your talk be new to the audience? Is the tone condescending or patronising?
- Are there any issues in which your audience will have a greater knowledge or expertise?
- Are there any controversial ideas or issues? How are the audience likely to react to these?
- What questions are likely to occur?

Calm your nerves

Try these tips to calm your nerves before your presentation:

- Remember a thorough preparation gives a sense of security.
- Take five minutes to relax before the talk. Relax your shoulders and breathe from the diaphragm. (See specific exercises in the chapter on *Effective Use of Voice*.)
- Concentrate on the audience. What questions might there be? Do they seem to be understanding?
- Remember the audience want you to succeed. They are on your side.

- Get plenty of sleep the night before.

Avoid the following common pitfalls

- *Confusing the audience by using jargon.* Always explain if you need to introduce unfamiliar terms.
- *Offending by being patronising.* Do not talk down to your audience.
- *Alienating your audience by using inappropriate remarks.* For example using 'deaf and dumb' instead of 'deaf' will offend many people.
- *Boring your audience.* Make sure your material is relevant and interesting.

Think positively

Despite the challenges of this type of presentation there are many positive aspects including the opportunity:

- To share knowledge and expertise. Your own and that in the audience.
- To do a PR job by telling people about your profession.
- To dispel any myths about your profession.
- To find out about other professions.
- To network by making contacts with other professionals.

Summary Points

- Consider the following factors:
    - The audience's background knowledge, experience and skills
    - The audience's attitude and perspective on the topic
    - The status of the audience in relation to the presenter
    - The language (particularly terminology) that are accessible for the audience.
- Research your audience thoroughly.

- Ask a friend or colleague from a similar background as your audience to listen to your presentation. Get feedback on the content and delivery.

- Calm your nerves by being thoroughly prepared. Take time before the presentation to relax. Remember the audience are on your side.

- Avoid common pitfalls such as being patronising, using inappropriate language, or using irrelevant material.

- Look upon your presentation as an opportunity to share information and learn about other professionals. This is the time to do a PR job on your profession.

Presentation Skills in Context
Lectures

The experienced clinician will be involved in training students both in their own or a related discipline. Tutoring is often 'on the job' with the student learning alongside the professional. Sometimes this role is extended to include formal lecturing. This section focuses on how you prepare and delivery such a lecture.

Preparation

Lectures differ from other presentations in a number of ways. First, the style of your delivery will be different. This is influenced by the characteristics of the audience. Students are familiar with the learning situation, and are therefore adept at tasks such as note taking, group discussions and other study skills. Second, the content of your lecture will be defined by pre-set parameters, such as the curriculum and the nature of student assessments. Both these factors will be tempered by the particular needs of each group of students, who will bring their own degree of experience, knowledge and skills.

One problem you might find as you start to prepare your lecture is that there seems to be insufficient time available to cover all the information. This is often the case when your material is very dear to your heart; for instance, if you are talking about your specialist subject or discussing your job. You therefore need to be ruthless about eliminating non-essential information.

The other point to consider is that the lecture is only part of the learning process for the student. Reading, reviewing notes and discussion help to consolidate and develop the student's understanding. This type of study immediately following a lecture also helps students remember information. It is estimated that students only remember half of what they hear in lectures, if no active use is made of the material (Gibbs 1981). Use the lecture to get your main points across, and prepare study guides for students to follow up information in depth.

Examples of active study include:

○ Set reading.

○ Providing a set of questions to focus students reading and note taking.

○ Diagrams or tables to be completed.

○ A problem solving task. For example, what aids and adaptions might be needed in the home for a patient with arthritic hips.

○ Data sets for applying newly learnt concepts.

○ True/false questionnaires. Students are provided with a statement which they have to mark as true or false. This helps provide them with feedback on their learning.

○ Detailed case studies provided for reference on a handout.

○ A practical task related to theory. For example, observation of mother's talking to their babies as a follow-up to a lecture on language development.

The structure of your lecture

Check that the structure of your lecture has a logical sequence, and builds on simple, familiar material before moving on to new and complex information. Here is an example of a lecture on the cardiovascular system:

Lecture on the cardiovascular system

Introduction: Living cells need food materials and oxygen. The circulatory system transports these materials to the cells of the body. The system consists of the heart (or pump) and blood vessels – arteries, veins and capillaries. There are two kinds of circulation – pulmonary and systemic.

Section I: Heart

Sub points – Position

Structure

Blood supply

Section 2: The conducting system of the heart

Sub points – Cardiac muscle

Pacemaker

Section 3: The cardiac cycle

Sub points – Systole/diastole

Heart rate

Section 4: Blood vessels

Subpoints – Arteries

Veins

Capillaries

Summary of the main points

Making your lecture interesting

Lectures make strenuous demands on students' concentration and listening skills. You need to plan for variety and novelty to stimulate interest and maintain attention (Gibbs, Habeshaw and Habeshaw 1989). Students are also more likely to remember information if they are involved in the lecture. Active listening promotes retention of information (Ellis and McClintock 1990). This involves students talking and acting upon what they are seeing and hearing.

Here are some examples of active listening activities:

- Discussing questions in pairs.
- A problem solving task for small groups.
- Completion of a gapped handout using video material. For example, noting the behaviour of a client while a case history is taken.
- Students design an information leaflet for clients using facts and figures provided in the lecture.
- A group discussion on how ideas can be applied to the workplace.
- Discussing provocative statements or opinions in small groups.
- Small groups draw up a summary of the key points from the lecture.

- Students are given a few minutes to check through their notes, or to swap notes with another student.

Making your explanations clearer

Lecturing is about teaching, and therefore explaining is a central strategy for any lecturer. These explanations need careful planning before the lecture. If you rely on your skills to ad lib on the day, you are likely to be vague and unclear. The first thing you need to do is decide whether you are describing What? How? or Why? (see a categorisation of explanations in *Giving Information* in the interview chapter).

It is useful to phrase your explanation as a what, how or why question. Once you have done this, you need to identify the hidden variables or key points within the explanation (Brown 1978).

Here are some examples of variables you would need to consider in giving the following explanations:

- *What is a chromosome?* – structure of cells, structure and composition of chromosomes, functions of chromosomes, sex chromosomes.
- *How to take a blood test?* – equipment, procedures, and precautions.
- *Why do people develop anaemia?* – definition, types of anaemia, gender differences, causes.

Explanations need some form of structure. They need a start and a finish. Main points need to be supported by examples and other forms of illustration. Here is a guide to the different devises you can use to make your explanations clearer.

Examples

Use examples to support your statements. They will be more effective if they are related to the audience's knowledge and experience. For instance, using the personal characteristics of the students to illustrate the sort of information carried by the genes of a chromosome.

Analogies

The use of an appropriate analogy can greatly improve understanding of abstract concepts. Consider this analogy used by an ENT surgeon giving a talk to parents of deaf children. He described how his wife enlists his help in shaking out the sheets after laundering. He asked the audience if they had noticed the small ripples that travel down the sheet as they are straightened. He then explained how these are similar to the waves created in air as sound travels to the ear. The simple analogy made use of an experience common to all of the audience.

Anecdotes

Telling a brief story can help lighten a lecture and improve understanding. Speakers also use more animated intonation when telling an anecdote, which will help provide some variety in delivery.

Quotes

These add interest as well as being useful to inform and explain points. The way that they are delivered can also add impact. For example, reading aloud from a newspaper suggests the information is up to date, newsworthy and therefore of importance.

Organising your lecture

Send the organiser an outline of your lecture. A reading list will also be appreciated. This can be given to the library, who will make sure that books are made available.

Do not assume that audio-visual aids will be available. Check with the organiser before hand, and stipulate any equipment that is essential. You will need to make arrangements with the college if you want to photocopy handouts.

Evaluating your lecture

Evaluation forms are a way of providing the lecturer with feedback. There are four areas that the student is usually asked to review:

- The content of the lecture
- The style of delivery
- The presentation skills of the lecturer
- Different aspects of course administration.

It depends on your aims and the requirements of the educational establishment whether you cover all of the areas or choose to concentrate on one or two.

Some of your aims might include the following:

- To evaluate your own performance (self monitoring allows you to improve your skills)

- To evaluate the content of the lecture (how appropriate did the students find the lecture material)
- To identify omissions in content
- To identify positive aspects of delivery or performance
- To audit the lecture (this will usually be part of an overall system of review within the educational establishment)
- To identify future needs of the students (useful for planning future courses).

Designing your form

There are a number of different ways of designing a form. Here are some common formats for eliciting information:

General headings

The student is provided with a general heading, such as 'Use of audio-visual aids', and asked to make comments. She is free to make observations about any aspect. The variety of responses that this method usually elicits makes it difficult to draw general conclusions. Some people are unsure how to respond when so little guidance is given on the type of responses required. So you can end up with lots of general comments, like 'OK' and 'good'. On the other hand it gives the opportunity for pertinent comments to arise on areas that you may not have anticipated.

Open questions

The student is asked to respond to a set of open questions. For example, 'What was the most useful part of the lecture?'. In this type of question the student is offered more direction, but responses can still be varied. Although it is the lecturer who has decided that 'usefulness' is an important criteria, it is left to the student to decide what parts of the lecture fulfilled this criteria.

Closed questions

These questions require the student to respond with a yes or no response to a direct question. For example, 'Did the lecturer provide a course outline?'. These types of question elicit specific information, but limit spontaneous comments. They are useful for obtaining information that may be needed for an audit of course administration. This would include items relating to the type of information provided to students, length of time for coursework to be returned and so on.

Statements

The student is provided with a set of statements. For example, 'Maintained my interest throughout the lecture'. The student is asked to respond to each statement by choosing a descriptor, such as – definitely, most of the time, about average, some of the time, or never. This approach provides more quantifiable information about a range of criteria. However, the lecturer is restricting comments to those aspects he or she has identified. There is also a tendency for people to choose an average rating. One solution to this problem is to add a supplementary section that asks for general comments. When devising this type of form, care needs to be taken that the variable can be measured by the scale. Is it possible to rate 'Stated the purpose of the lecture' on the above scale?

Indirect questions

You may want to use indirect questions to elicit information. For example, the closed question 'Was the style of delivery boring?' could be replaced with 'Did you find it hard to concentrate?'. The statement 'Stimulates my interest in the subject' could be replaced by 'Were you inspired to read more on the subject?'

An alternative approach is to ask your students to design an evaluation form. This will provide you with an insight into what the student values in a lecture and a lecturer.

A colleague had these responses when she asked her students for comments:

- Flexibility by the lecturer
- Someone who knows their subject
- Well organised structure
- Enthusiasm
- Video material related to theoretical background
- Opportunity to work in small groups and feed back conclusions to whole class
- Time allowed for questions
- Lecturer willing to discuss the subject.

Action Points

Compare the examples of evaluation questionnaires in Figures 4.6., 4.7. and 4.8.

Evaluation questionnaire

Date of Lecture: 20th June 1995

Title: **'Hearing Tests for Infants'**

Please comment on the following aspects of today's lecture. This feedback is useful for planning future lectures on this subject. Thank you.

1. Content of Lecture:

2. Delivery of Lecture (pace, clarity, interest):

3. Use of audio-visual aids:

4. Any other comments:

5. Are there any topics that you felt were not included?

6. Please write your suggestions for future topics or add any other comments:

Figure 4.6

Evaluation questionnaire

Date of Lecture: 20th June 1995

1. How valuable was the lecture?

    very valuable – much learnt   ☐

    good value – learnt quite alot   ☐

    some value   ☐

    little value   ☐

2. What was the most valuable part of the lecture?

3. Was there any part of the lecture that had too much time?

4. Was there any part of the lecture that needed more time?

5. Should anything have been included which was not? If so, what?

6. How well was the lecture presented?

    very well   ☐

    well   ☐

    satisfactory   ☐

    poorly   ☐

7. Please write your suggestions for future topics or add any other comments:

Figure 4.7

Evaluation questionnaire

Title: 'Hearing Tests for Infants'

Date of Lecture: 20th June 1995

Please circle the appropriate rating for the various aspects of the above course.

1 poor   2 adequate   3 good   4 very good   5 excellent

Delivery:

Pace of presentation	1 2 3 4 5
Overall structure	1 2 3 4 5
Logic and clarity of explanations	1 2 3 4 5
Encouragement of student participation	1 2 3 4 5
Quality of handouts	1 2 3 4 5

Content:

Relevance to students	1 2 3 4 5
Key points emphasised	1 2 3 4 5
Amount of information adequate	1 2 3 4 5
Appropriate level	1 2 3 4 5
Use of examples and illustrations	1 2 3 4 5

Presentation:

Regular eye-contact maintained	1 2 3 4 5
Effective use of gesture	1 2 3 4 5
Rapport with students	1 2 3 4 5
Communication skills	1 2 3 4 5

Audio-visual aids:

Clarity	1 2 3 4 5
Appropriateness	1 2 3 4 5
Variety	1 2 3 4 5

Please write any other comments:

Thank you

Figure 4.8

(1) How will the information yielded differ with each form?

(2) What are the advantages and disadvantages of each format?

(3) Which style of form would you like to complete?

(4) Which forms give you specific ideas about improving the lecture?

(5) Check each form and decide whether questions are phrased negatively or positively? This can have an impact on the type of responses you receive.

(6) When designing your own evaluation form think about the following questions:

- What is the purpose of the evaluation form?

- What areas do you want to cover?

- Do you want a rating system?

- How will the information be used?

- How much time is available for

(1) the students to complete the form

(2) you to summarise the findings.

Summary Points

- The experienced clinician will be involved in training students both in their own or a related discipline. Sometimes this role is extended to include formal lecturing.

- The style of delivery and content of the lecture are influenced by the characteristics of the audience and the restrictions of curriculum and assessment.

- The lecture will only cover the key points. Further learning takes place through active study by the students.

- The most common format for a lecture involves dividing the information into several broad categories or themes. These form the main sections of the lecture. Each of which consists of several points that support the main theme.

- Use activities that promote active listening. Students are more likely to remember if they talk and act upon what they see and hear.

- Plan your explanations carefully. They need to have a structure that includes a start, a statement of the main points and a finish.

- Decide whether your explanation is a what, how or why question. Identify the key points within your explanation.

- Support your explanations with examples, analogies, anecdotes and quotes.

- Use student questionnaires to evaluate your lectures.

Presentation Skills in Context
Selling your Service

'Selling' has previously been an alien concept to most health professionals. Following the National Health Service (NHS) reforms and the introduction of the market place ideology to health care, many managers are now involved in negotiating service contracts. Although you may feel you know very little about marketing or selling, each of us engages in some form of persuasion every day. This may be deciding who picks the children up from school or allocating tasks to team members. Selling your service will involve some of these everyday skills of persuasion.

One form of persuasion is the promotional presentation. This section looks specifically at how you can market your service through this type of presentation.

There are three main points you need to think about when preparing your presentation. These are:

what?

who?

how?

- ◦ What are you selling?
- ◦ Who is your buyer?
- ◦ How will you sell?

What are you selling?

Use the format of your service contract as a guide when preparing the content of your talk. A contract between a provider and a purchaser will have three elements. These are price, quantity and quality (Øvretveit 1994). Quantity refers to the demand for your service and your responses to these demands. Quality may be defined in a variety of ways. The resources used to meet these demands for your service are one measure, for example the number of specialist health visitors required for under fives with special needs. Standards of care or measures of quality assurance is another, for example the length of waiting lists for a first appointment for chiropody. A third measure of quality is outcomes, for example the number of children receiving vaccinations. Price refers to the cost of providing this service plus any spare capacity you might want to build into the agreement.

These elements are interdependent; each one relates to the other. Øvretveit (1994) refers to this relationship as the contract triangle. A change in one element affects the other two. So, an increase in quality means either an increase in price or a decrease in quantity.

You need to know exactly what you are selling and be able to clearly convey this to the purchaser. The first step is to identify the demand for your service, and how you intend to meet this demand. You then need to draw up a comprehensive description of the features of your service. Here are some questions to help your preparation:

✧ **Who is the target client group?**
Be specific. This is evidence of the demand for your service. Detail relevant medical conditions, age range, gender, and the estimated number of clients who would benefit from the service.

✧ **What is the purpose of your service?**
Is it an assessment only service? Do you provide out-patient treatment? Think about the results or outcomes of your service.

✧ **What type of service are you offering?**
Acute; out-patient; domicillary; preventative medicine; or health promotion.

✧ **Where will your service be delivered?**
A specialised centre; in the home of the client; a community clinic; hospital.

✧ **How often?**
Is it a monthly clinic? Service on demand?

Next you need to think about the quantity element of the contract triangle. What is your response to the demand for your service? Provide information on either the numbers of clients (output) or the amount of staff time (input).

There has been a shift in focus regarding funding in the NHS. The emphasis has moved from staffing levels to the idea of the end product. You may therefore want to concentrate on output in your presentation, although of course input will affect your final price.

Can you define the quality of your service? One measure of quality is the type of staff, or in other words the human resources, needed to provide the service. You may offer a specialist service that is not widely available elsewhere. If so, you would focus on this aspect during your presentation.

In addition you need to outline your quality assurance systems. Purchasers want to know how you are measuring quality. Check the systems used by the purchasers. Are they similar to yours? If so, this can be highlighted in your presentation as a benefit.

The outcomes from your service are crucial. They are the justification for the provision of your service. These need to be documented with care.

How will you sell your service? or the art of persuasion

Selling always involves a large measure of persuasion. You are persuading the purchaser that they need this type of service. You also want them to choose you to deliver it. To negotiate a sale you need to be able to understand the buyer's perspective, anticipate objections and tailor your presentation to their needs.

Who is your buyer?

Study your potential purchasers. The key to effective selling is researching your customer thoroughly (Heylin 1991). Find out about the culture of the organisation. Are they expanding or contracting their services? What are their priorities for health care provision? Think about why the purchasers would want your service. Successful marketing involves matching your service with the needs of the buyer (Randall 1994).

Since the patient's charter, users of health care services are more knowledgeable about getting services. This creates pressure on purchasers if there is a restricted service in the client's health area for a particular specialism. Use this to your advantage by alerting purchasers to potential problems. An increase in the number of complaints can be used positively as an indicator of need.

Organising the team presentation

The presentation is likely to be a team effort that will include colleagues, and other professionals if your service is part of an integrated service; for example, a rehabilitation unit for stroke victims. Team presentations require co-ordination and careful preparation. The first step is to decide the different roles that people will play in the procedures. Elect one person to take responsibility for co-ordinating the arrangements. This includes organising meetings and following up progress with individual team members.

You will also need to decide who in the group will make the actual presentation. It is important to select speakers on the basis of ability, not on seniority or the desire to 'include everybody'.

Preparing the presentation

Preparation involves the presentation team in meeting regularly to discuss the aims and content of the talk. Once the general outline has been agreed, individual speakers can prepare their initial notes. These need to be discussed at a further meeting either with the team co-ordinator or the group as a whole. Once the speakers have their final draft, the team need to review the complete presentation. Each member will need to run through the content of their talk. It will be difficult to get an overall impression until all the presenters are heard and seen together. This will provide an opportunity to check for errors, duplication, omissions, ambiguities or contradictions. Any difficulties with timing and continuity can also be sorted out at this stage. A final dress rehearsal is essential. Aim to end on a high note. Perhaps a glass of wine for everybody!

Deciding on the format

Start with something that will get the audience interested. This could be the number of complaints about the lack of service, or an account of a day in the life of one of your clients. The former addresses a possible need for the purchaser to reduce complaints, the latter provides information about the needs of the people your service will be helping. Your choice will depend on the motivations and needs of your purchaser.

The aim of the presentation is to sell the service. Giving a point by point description of your service is unlikely to achieve this, no matter how excellent it is. Start by focusing attention on the needs of the purchasers (Wilder 1990). These will have been identified during your research of the purchasing body.

Listen to the feedback you get from the audience. Do not be afraid to ask questions to find out exactly what the purchaser wants.

The next part of the presentation will be a description of your service. This needs to be framed in a way that will answer the unspoken questions you think will be in the minds of the audience. These might include, 'Why do we need a specialist service?', 'How much will it cost?', 'What measures will be taken to ensure that the contract is fulfilled?' Try to establish the likely objections and prepare responses that answer them in full.

Exploit the marketable benefits of your service and make these clear in your presentation. At the end of the presentation the audience should have all the information they need in order to make a decision about purchasing.

Delivering your message

The way that you deliver the presentation will send covert messages to the purchaser. Make sure these are positive ones. Will the audience be impressed with the efficiency of your service, if you forget your overheads or mix up your slides? Duplication or differences of opinion between co-presenters suggests at best a lack of communication, at worst disharmony. Positive messages to convey are:

- Unity
- Cohesion
- Efficiency
- Enthusiasm
- Dynamic management
- Organisation
- Commitment.

This is not the time for presenters to be competing for attention. Decide who will deal with queries and stick to this agreement. Provide the audience with the names and job titles of all the presentation team, and include information about their role in the presentation.

The way that you communicate is part of the selling process. Use open and friendly body language during the talk, and give lots of eye contact. Talk about your service as if it was already contracted to the purchasers.

Using audio-visual aids

Choose one member to take charge of audio-visual aids. This person has responsibility for preparing the material and taking an overview of the content. It also ensures that the style and format of visuals will be consistent between presenters. This communicates a sense of cohesion and reinforces the idea of a service rather than a group of individuals. On the day of the presentation this person can supervise the set-up of equipment and assist in delivering a smooth performance.

Use visuals to get your message across quickly and efficiently. If possible, use colour as this is more persuasive than black and white. Remember a title can be used to sell an idea. Compare 'Waiting lists for 1995–1996' with

'Waiting lists cut by 50%'. A graphic display of the actual fall in numbers can support the title, with exact figures supplied on a hand-out.

Make sure your service logo is prominent on all your visuals and hand-outs. An enlarged image of your logo can be placed alongside the title on your first visual. Use your logo on the interleaving pages between prepared flip chart sheets. It can be placed in the top right hand corner on acetates and slides.

Your last visual is the most important. Think carefully about the final message you want to leave in the minds of the audience. It helps if you can link it with the idea in your first visual or opening statement.

Summary Points

- Know what you are selling.
- Research your purchaser thoroughly.
- Focus on the needs of the purchaser, and expand on the benefits your service offers.
- Elect a team leader to co-ordinate the planning and preparation of the presentation.
- Select speakers on the basis of merit and not seniority.
- Choose one team member to prepare and supervise the use of audio-visual aids.
- Use your visual aids to help sell your message. Rehearse your presentation in full before the big day.
- Remember how you deliver the presentation is just as important as what you say.
- Be a good listener. Ask the audience questions and find out all the details of any objections.
- Make sure the purchasers have all the information they need to make a decision.

Presentation Skills in Context
Presenting your Research

There are two things about research that make it an easier topic to present than others. One is its novelty to the audience. Research is about new ideas and events. The second is your enthusiasm for the subject. These two different aspects will stimulate the audience's interest and maintain their attention.

As with other presentations, your style of delivery will depend on your aims and your target audience. Shared vocabulary, assumed knowledge and interest in the subject will differ greatly between an audience of researchers and an audience of lay people. This needs to be taken into account when planning your presentation.

The format of your presentation

Your title

What is the title of your presentation? Some research titles sound very dry. Think of ways to make yours more interesting. Use humour or a provocative statement. Even phrasing your title as a question can make a difference.

Decide whether you will give a hint of your results in the title. This will wet the audience's appetite. Alternatively keep the audience in suspense by building up to the results during the presentation. This way you can play the 'will they, won't they angle'.

Introductions

Introduce yourself to the audience with some brief background details. Follow this with some basic information about the purpose of your research, and more specifically your experimental question. Get your audience interested in what you are going to say, by talking about your reasons for choosing the research. This might include the importance of your research to health care, or the way in which your study overcame previous difficulties in research methodology.

Help orientate the audience to the topic by giving a brief overview of related studies. The emphasis is on brief. Avoid giving too much detail.

The content of your talk

The main body of the talk will include information on your methodology, results, and the conclusions you have drawn from your findings. Instead of regurgitating your project like a dissertation, tell a story. The detective who solves a problem. The explorer who makes a journey of discovery. The intrepid traveller who overcomes various difficulties to reach the journey's end. You do not have take on the persona, or even refer to explorers, travellers or detectives. The similarity is in how you structure your talk. For example, describing how you solved the problem of finding matched subjects.

The essential item of interest to the audience is the results of your research. You need to think carefully about the best way to present your material in the limited time available. Select the most relevant aspects, and use graphics to convey information quickly and simply. (See the section below for ideas on presenting your material.)

Plan your time to allow for an adequate discussion of the results, and be prepared to respond to queries from the audience. State your evaluation clearly, relating the findings back to your original hypothesis or experimental question. This will draw your presentation together for the audience. You may want to support your arguments with references to previous research findings. Alternatively you may want to highlight how your research contradicts previously held views. Be careful not to swamp the audience with numerous references to the literature. Your findings are the main focus.

During your conclusion reiterate the main points of your evaluation. Give a brief indication of how the information obtained from the study can be applied clinically, or describe its significance to theory.

Your presentation is likely to prompt questions from the audience. This is all part of sharing and debating research. See the chapter on *Delivering Content* for tips on how to deal with questions.

Preparing visual displays for numerical information

Visual presentation of numerical information needs to be accurate, but simple enough for the audience to understand and assimilate quickly.

The most common forms of visual display are:

- ○ Tables

- ○ Bar charts
- ○ Pie charts
- ○ Line graphs.

Tables

Tables can be a complete record of your original data or a summary of the essential information. Complex tables are best presented on a handout. Tables for presentation on a slide or acetate need to be simple, with only the most relevant details included. Use the minimum number of rows and columns. Show your units of measurement, and round off your figures if possible.

DESIGN TIPS

- ◊ Choose symbols or icons for use in tables carefully. Do they already have a universal meaning? For instance, a tick is seen as positive; this type of cross 'X' suggests an error; this type of cross '+' implies addition.
- ◊ The audience will be used to seeing figures listed down a page, so place them in columns rather than rows.

Bar charts

These are a simple but effective way to display information. They are suitable for nominal level data, where subjects or items are classified into categories. There are different types of bar chart that include vertical, horizontal, multiple and proportional.

Vertical bar charts

Each category is represented by a vertical bar, the height of which relates to the numerical value of that category. Use vertical bar charts to show comparisons between categories.

Figure 4.9 shows the number of chiropody appointments at one health centre. These are classified according to the year in which they occurred. This way the number of appointments can be compared over a three year period. The chart clearly illustrates an increase in chiropody appointments.

DESIGN TIPS

- ◊ Display time on the horizontal axis.
- ◊ Indent the first bar so that it is set away from the y axis.

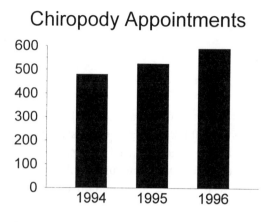

Figure 4.9 Vertical bar chart

Horizontal bar charts

Each category is represented by a horizontal bar. The length of the bar representing the numerical value of the data. These bar charts show comparisons between categories at a single point in time.

Figure 4.10 shows the chiropody, dental and speech therapy appointments at a health centre. The chart allows the monthly figures to be compared.

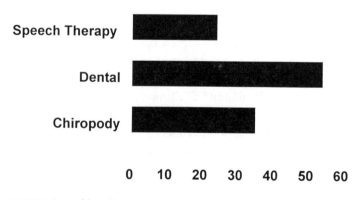

Figure 4.10 Horizontal bar chart

DESIGN TIP

◊ Write the names of the categories instead of having a y axis.

Multiple bar charts

Multiple or compound bar charts show comparisons between related sets of categories.

In Figure 4.11 the number of beds in different medical specialities is compared over a three year period. This shows a decline in medical and surgical beds, whilst neuro beds have remained constant.

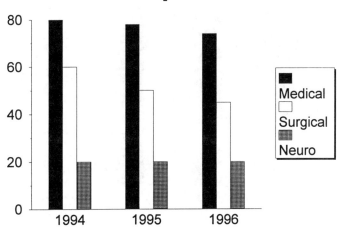

Figure 4.11 Multiple bar chart

DESIGN TIPS

◊ Use different colours or shading to provide a contrast between each bar.

◊ Use the same colour or shading for each category, so they are instantly recognisable.

Proportional bar charts

These charts are also known as stratified, stacked or component bar charts. They show the division of the whole into its relative proportions. Each bar represents the whole, and each segment part of that whole. It is possible to make comparisons between both the whole and the constituent parts.

Figure 4.12 shows the number of nursing, medical and administrative staff employed in a health centre over a three year period. It is possible to compare the whole, or total number of staff, over that time. We can see from the chart that staffing increased in 1995, and then dropped in 1996 below the level of 1994. The constituent parts, or individual staff groupings, can also be compared. The chart shows an increase in medical and administrative staff over the three year period. Nursing after rising slightly in 1995, fell below the 1994 level the following year.

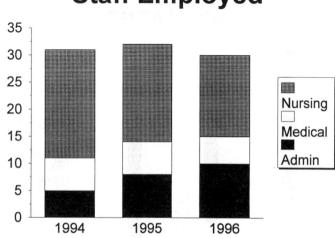

Figure 4.12 Proportional bar chart

DESIGN TIPS

◊ Use colours or shading to provide a contrast between each component of the bar.

◊ Use the same colour to represent the same component on different bars.

GENERAL HINTS FOR BAR CHARTS

◊ Write labels across the page and not down the side of the graph. (Otherwise the audience will be twisting and turning their heads to read the labels.)

◊ Keep information to a minimum. The audience will have difficulty in assimilating information from graphs that have more than five bars.

◊ Solid bars are easier to see than an outline. It also helps if the bars are wider than the interleaving spaces.

Pie charts

Pie charts have an immediate and powerful visual impact. They are suitable for nominal level data, where subjects or items are classified into categories. Use them to show what proportions make up a whole, rather than specific details of figures. Avoid using pie charts to compare sets of data, as this tends to be less effective visually.

Figure 4.13 illustrates the staff groupings within a community health trust.

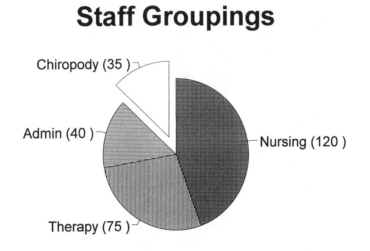

Figure 4.13 Pie chart

DESIGN TIPS

◊ Limit segments to a maximum of six.

◊ Start segments at the twelve o'clock position.

◊ Sequence segments in order of size.

◊ Colour or shade segments and use a key.

◊ Explode out segments you want to highlight. Make sure they are at the twelve o'clock position.

Line graphs

Use line graphs for data at ordinal or interval level. They are useful for showing either consistency or changes over time.

Figure 4.14 shows the record of weight loss for two clients following separate diets.

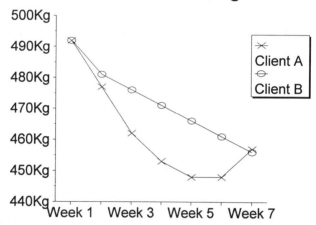

Figure 4.14 Line chart

DESIGN TIPS

◊ Keep to a maximum of three lines per graph.

◊ Use colour to differentiate between lines.

◊ Use a bright colour or bold line to emphasise the most important line.

Preparing visuals

Follow these rules when preparing your visuals:

○ Keep it simple

○ Make it clear

○ Give it impact.

Keep it simple

Complex images are difficult for the audience to assimilate quickly. Extract the essential information and display it in a simpler form. You may need to break down a complex graph into two or three simpler ones. Avoid having too many graphs or charts on one visual. As a rule, three is the absolute maximum.

There is a limit to the amount of information that can be shown on an overhead or slide without losing legibility. The more text and numerals on the visual, the more difficult it will be to enlarge these to a size that is readable at a distance. So keep details to a minimum.

Make it clear

Your visual needs to be instantly understandable. Use labels to help the audience interpret the material. Keep these simple and make sure they are readable. Words and numerals should go across the page. Avoid writing labels vertically up the side of a graph, or along the spokes of a pie chart. Otherwise the audience will have to stand on their head to read some of the titles.

Colour and shading can also help the audience make sense of the information. Use highlighting to focus the audience's attention on key figures, lines, or segments. Emphasise text by marking it in bold or using a bright colour. On black and white visuals use a solid line for the most important information. In a table a whole row or column can be highlighted by surrounding it by a box.

Give it Impact

Think about what you want to show with your graphics. What is the message of your visual? Use visuals that show what your results mean, not just the numbers.

Simple information can be displayed as pictograms. These are pictures that represent the data. For example, the incidence of heart attack in different geographical populations could be represented by broken hearts placed on a map. Each symbol denoting a set figure like 1000 people. Using the colour red would give the pictogram even greater impact. Pictograms are useful to show trends, but are less precise than other graphics.

Always supply handouts that duplicate the information supplied on a visual. Talk the audience through the details. Never assume they will see the obvious.

Presenting Your Research Checklist

☐ The title of your presentation will arouse the interest of the audience

Introduction

☐ The aims of your research are clearly explained

☐ You have stated your experimental question or hypothesis

☐ Your opening statement includes your reasons for doing the research

☐ Other related studies have been briefly mentioned

The content of your talk

Your design has been fully explained and includes:

☐ Details of subjects (if appropriate)

☐ Selection criteria for subjects (if appropriate)

☐ A description of the materials used in the research

☐ A description of the methodology

☐ An outline of the scoring system or method of analysis

☐ The names of the statistical test(s) used in the research

☐ The rationale for the choice of the statistical test and level of significance

Your results:

☐ The main findings are summarised

☐ Your results are displayed visually

☐ Your graphics are clear and simple

☐ Detailed information is available on handouts

Evaluation of your research:

☐ The findings are clearly explained

☐ The results are related to the original hypothesis

☐ The significance of the results is discussed

Your summary includes:

☐ Suggestions for future research

☐ Practical applications of your research

Delivery:

☐ You have developed an interesting format for delivering your presentation.

Response to questions:

☐ You have prepared explanations to account for any inconsistencies or unexpected findings

Summary Points

○ Research by nature is novel, and therefore has an intrinsic attraction for the audience.

○ Avoid presenting a dissertation. Make a story. Present a problem that needs to be solved or describe a series of discoveries.

○ The main body of the talk will contain information on your methodology, results and conclusions.

○ The results will form the core of your presentation. Use graphics to convey them quickly and simply. Choose a display that suits your data.

○ Graphics need to be simple, clear and have impact. Additional details can be provided on handouts.

○ Offer an evaluation of your study. Relate this to your hypothesis, and to other related studies.

○ Give a brief indication of how your study can be applied clinically, or describe its significance to theory.

References

Anstey, E. (1962) *Committees: How They Work and How to Work Them.* London: Allen and Unwin.

Argyle, M. (1978) *The Psychology of Interpersonal Behaviour.* Harmondsworth, Middlesex: Penguin Books.

Argyle, M. (1988) *Bodily Communication.* London: Routledge.

Argyle, M. and Cook, M. (1976) *Gaze and Mutual Gaze.* Cambridge: Cambridge University Press.

Argyle, M. and Dean, J. (1965) 'Eye-contact, distance and affiliation.' *Sociometry 28*, 289–304.

Armstrong, S.L. (1984) 'What some concepts might not be.' *Cognition 13*, 263–308.

Arvey, R. and Campion, J. (1984) 'Person perception in the employment interview.' In M. Cook (ed) *Issues in Person Perception.* London: Methuen.

Baken, R.J. (1991) 'An overview of laryngeal function for voice production.' In R.T. Sataloff, *Professional Voice: The Science and Art of Clinical Care.* New York: Raven Press.

Bales, R.F. (1970) *Personality and Interpersonal Behavior.* New York: Holt, Rinehart and Winston.

Berne, E. (1964) *Games People Play.* Harmondsworth, Middlesex: Penguin.

Binsted, D. (1986) *Developments in Interpersonal Skills Training.* Aldershot, Hampshire: Gower Publishing.

Bligh, D. (1983) *What's the use of Lectures?* Harmondsworth, Middlesex: Penguin.

Bond, T. (1986) *Games for Social and Life Skills.* London: Hutchinson.

Borden, G.J. and Harris, K.S. (1980) *Speech Science Primer.* Baltimore: The Williams and Wilkins Co.

Breakwell, G.M. (1990) *Interviewing.* Leicester: The British Psychological Society and Routledge.

Brown, G. (1978) *Lecturing and Explaining.* London: Methuen.

Bull, P. (1983) *Body Movement and Interpersonal Communication.* Chichester, Sussex: John Wiley and Sons.

Bull, P. (1987) *Posture and Gesture.* Oxford: Pergamon.

Bull, P. and Connelly, G. (1985) 'Body movement and emphasis in speech.' *Journal of Non-Verbal Behaviour 9*, 169–87.

Bunch, M. (1982) *Dynamics of the Singing Voice.* New York: Springer-Verlag Wien.

Bunch, M. (1995) *Succeed at Work and Play.* Person to Person Audio Cassettes.

Burnard, P. (1992) *Effective Communication Skills for Health Professionals.* London: Chapman and Hall.

Butler, P.E. (1992) *Self-Assertion for Women.* San Francisco: Harper.

Clare, A. (1991) 'Developing communication and interviewing skills.' In R. Corney, *Developing Communication and Counselling Skills in Medicine.* London: Routledge.

Cohen, W.I. (1983) 'Establishing effective parent/patient communication.' In M. King, L. Novak and C. Citrenbaum, *Irresistible Communication: Creative Skills for the Health Professional.* London: W.B. Saunders.

Cohen-Cole, S.A. and Bird, J. (1991) 'Function 1: gathering data to understand the patient.' In S.A. Cohen-Cole (ed) *The Medical Interview: The Three-Function Approach.* St.Louis: Mosby Year Book.

Cook, M. (1970) 'Experiments on orientation and proxemics.' *Human Relations 23,* 61–76.

Corney, R. (ed) (1991) *Developing Communication and Counselling Skills in Medicine.* London: Routledge.

Council for the Advancement of Communication with Deaf People: Directory '94 – '95, Pelaw House, School of Education, University of Durham.

Croner (1985) *Croner's Guide to Interviews.* London: Croner Publications.

Darley, F.L., Aronson, A.E. and Brown, J.R. (1975) *Motor Speech Disorders.* London: W.B. Saunders Co.

Denes, P.B. and Pinson, E.N. (1973) *The Speech Chain.* London: Anchor Books.

Deuchar, M. (1984) *British Sign Language.* London: Routledge.

Dickson, A. (1982) *A Woman in Your Own Right.* London: Quartet Books.

Dickson, D.A., Hargie, O. and Morrow, N.C. (1989) *Communication Skills Training for Health Professionals.* London: Chapman and Hall.

Duncan, S. and Fiske, D.W. (1977) *Face-face Interaction: Research Methods and Theory.* New Jersey: Lawrence Erlbaum Associates.

Ekman, P. (1982) *Emotion in the Human Face,* (2nd edition). Cambridge: Cambridge University Press.

Ekman, P. (1985) *Telling Lies.* New York: Norton.

Ekman, P. and Friesen, W.V. (1969) 'The repertoire of non-verbal behaviour: Categories, origins, usage, and coding.' *Semiotica 1,* 49–98.

Ekman, P. and Friesen, W.V. (1982) 'Felt, false, and miserable smiles.' *Journal of Non-Verbal Behavior 6,* 238–52.

Ellis, R. and McClintock, A. (1990) *If You Take My Meaning*. London: Edward Arnold.

Fawcus, R. (1986) 'The physiology of phonation.' In M. Fawcus (ed) *Voice Disorders and their Management*, (2nd edition). London: Chapman and Hall.

Forsyth, P. (1995) *Making Successful Presentations*. London: Sheldon Press.

Freeburn, R. (1993) 'Words, words, words.' *Modern Management 7*, 13–14.

Freeburn, R. (1994) 'Communication with a difference.' *Network* (Winter 93/94) 41–42.

Freedman, N. and Hoffman, S.P. (1967) 'Kinetic behaviour in altered clinical states:Approach to objective analysis of motor behaviour during interviews.' *Perceptual and Motor Skills 24*, 527–39.

Frick, R.W. (1985) 'Communicating emotion: The role of prosodic features.' *Psychological Bulletin 97*, 412–29.

Gahagan, J. (1975) *Essential Psychology*. London: Methuen.

Gask, L. (1991) 'Identifying emotional and psychosocial problems.' In R. Corney, *Developing Communication and Counselling Skills*. London: Routledge.

Gibbs, G. (1981) Twenty terrible reasons for lecturing. Paper No 8. Birmingham: Standing Conference in Educational Development.

Gibbs, G. (1992) Teaching More Students: Number 2 Lecturing to more students. The Polytechnics and Colleges Funding Council.

Gibbs, G., Habeshaw, S. and Habeshaw, T. (1989) *53 Interesting Things to do in your Lectures*. Bristol: Technical and Educational Services.

Gilroy, J. and Holliday, P.L. (1982) *Basic Neurology*. London: Collier Macmillan.

Gimson, A.C. (1980) *An Introduction to the Pronunciation of English*, (3rd edition). London: Edward Arnold.

Goodworth, C.T. (1979) *Effective Interviewing for Employment Selection*. London: Business Books.

Graham, J. and Argyle, M. (1975) 'A cross-cultural study of the communication of extra-verbal meaning by gestures.' *International Journal of Psychology 10*, 56–67.

Gratus, J. (1990) *Give and Take: A Practical Guide to Making the Most of Meetings*. London: BBC Books.

Hall, E.T. (1966) *The Hidden Dimension*. New York: Doubleday.

Hampton, J.R., Harrison, M.J.E., Mitchell, J.R.A., Pritchard, J.S. and Seymour, C. (1975) 'Relative contributions of history taking, physical examination and laboratory investigation to diagnosis and management of medical outpatients.' *British Medical Journal ii*, 486–9.

Hargie, O., Saunders, C. and Dickson, D. (1994) *Social Skills in Interpersonal Communication*, (3rd edition). London: Routledge.

Harrigan, J.A., Oxman, T.E. and Rosenthal, R. (1985) 'Rapport expressed through nonverbal behavior.' *Journal of Nonverbal Behavior 9*, 2, 95–110.

Hauge, M. (1989) *Writing Screenplays that Sell*. London: Elm Tree Books.

Herriot, P. (1989) *Recruitment in the 90s*. London: Institute of Personnel Management.

Heylin, A. (1991) *Putting it Across*. London: Michael Joseph.

Hirano, M. (1981) *Clinical Examination of Voice*. New York: Springer-Verlag Wien.

Hunt, N. (1992) *How to Conduct Staff Appraisals – A Practical Handbook for Every Manager Today*. Plymouth: How to Books Ltd.

Huntington, D. (1987) *Social Skills and General Medical Practice*. London: Allen and Unwin.

Ingram, I.M., Timbury, G.C. and Mowbray, R.M. (1981) *Notes on Psychiatry*. Edinburgh: Churchill Livingstone.

Izard, C.E. (1977) *Human Emotions*. New York: Plenum.

Izard, C.E. (1978) 'On the development of emotions and emotion-cognition relationships in infancy.' In M.A. Lewis and L.A. Rosenbaum (eds) *The Development of Affect*. New York: Plenum.

Jay, A. (1993) *Effective Presentation*. London: Pitman Publishing.

Jourard, S.M. (1966) 'An exploratory study of body-accessibility.' *British Journal of Social and Clinical Psychology 46*, 130–138.

Kaplan, H.M. (1960) *Anatomy and Physiology of Speech*. London: McGraw-Hill.

King, M., Novik, L. and Citrenbaum, C. (1983) *Irresistible Communication* (Creative skills for the health professional). London: W.B. Saunders.

Kleinke, C.L. (1986) 'Gaze and eye-contact: A research review.' *Psychological Bulletin 100*, 78–100.

Knapp, M.L., Hart, R., Friedrich, G. and Schulman, G. (1973) 'The rhetoric of goodbye: Verbal and non-verbal correlates of human leave-taking.' *Speech Monographs 40*, 182–198.

Koontz, H. and O'Donnell, C. (1984) *Management*. New York: McGraw-Hill.

Krasner, L. (1958) 'Studies of the conditioning of verbal behaviour.' *Psychological Bulletin 55*, 148–170.

L'Armand, K. (1984) 'Preferences in patterns of eye-contact in India.' *Journal of Social Psychology 122*, 137–138.

Lamb, W. and Watson, E. (1979) *Body Code*. London: Routledge and Kegan Paul.

Ley, P. (1982) 'Understanding, memory, satisfaction and compliance.' *British Journal of Clinical Psychology 21*, 241–254.

Ley, P. (1988) *Communicating with Patients*. London: Croom Helm.

Ley, P., Bradshaw, P.W., Kincey, J.A. and Atherton, S.T. (1976) 'Increasing patients' satisfaction with communications.' *British Journal of Social Clinical Psychology 15*, 403–413.

Locke, M. (1980) *How to Run Committees and Meetings.* London: The MacMillan Press.

Maddux, R.B. (1987) *Effective Performance Appraisals.* London: Kogan Page.

Maguire, P. (1991) 'Managing difficult communication tasks.' In R. Corney (ed) *Developing Communication and Counselling Skills in Medicine.* London: Routledge.

Martin, S. (1987) *Working with Dysphonics.* Bicester: Oxford.

Matarazzo, J.D., Wiens, A.N. and Saslow, G. (1965) 'Studies in interview speech behavior.' In L. Krasner and L. Ullman (eds) *Research in Behavior Modification: New Developments and Implications.* New York: Holt, Rinehart and Winston.

Mehrabian, A. (1972) *Nonverbal Communication.* Chicago: Aldine-Atherton.

Morris, D. (1978) *Manwatching.* London: Cape.

Murphy, C.M. and Messer, D.J. (1977) 'Mothers, infants and pointing: A study of gesture.' In R.E. Schaffer (ed) *Studies in Mother–infant Interaction.* London: Academic Press.

Myerscough, P.R. (1989) *Talking with Patients – A Basic Clinical Skill.* Oxford: Oxford Medical Publications.

Newell, R. (1994) *Interviewing Skills for Nurses and other Health Care Professionals.* London: Routledge.

Noesjirwan, J. (1978) 'A rule-based analysis of cultural differences in social behaviour: Indonesia and Australia.' *International Journal of Psychology 13*, 305–316.

Northern, J.L. and Downs, M.P. (1974) *Hearing in Children.* Maryland: The Williams and Wilkins Co.

Pedler, M., Burgoyne, J. and Boydell, T. (1994) *A Manager's Guide to Self-Development*, (3rd edition). London: McGraw-Hill.

Open University Coping with Crisis Group (1987) *Running Workshops: A Guide for Trainers in the Helping Professions.* London: Croom Helm.

Ovretveit, J. (1994) 'Expand your service by contracting.' *CSLT Bulletin* March 7–10.

Pendleton, D., Schofield, T., Tate, P. and Havelock, P. (1984) *The Consultation – An Approach to Teaching and Learning.* Oxford: Oxford University Press.

Perkins, W.H. and Kent, R.D. (1986) *Textbook of Functional Anatomy of Speech, Language and Hearing.* London: Taylor and Francis.

Porritt, L. (1984) *Communication Choices for Nurses*. Edinburgh: Churchill Livingstone.

Randall, G. (1994) *Effective Marketing*. London: Routledge.

Randell, G., Packard, P. and Slater, J. (1984) *Staff Appraisal: A First Step to Effective Leadership*, (3rd Edition). London: Institute of Personnel Management.

Rees, W.D. (1991) *The Skills of Management*, (3rd edition). London: Routledge.

Riseborough, M.G. (1981) 'Physiographic gestures as decoding facilitators:Three experiments exploring a neglected facet of communication.' *Journal of NonVerbal Behavior 5*, 173–183.

Roberts, C. (1985) *The Interviewing Game*. London: BBC Books.

Rogers, W. (1978) 'The contribution of kinesic illustrators toward the comprehension of verbal behavior within utterances.' *Human Communication Research 5*, 54–62.

Rosenshine, B. (1968) *Teaching Behaviour and Student Achievement*. Windsor: National Foundation for Educational Research in England and Wales.

Sataloff, R.T. (1991) *Professional Voice: The Science and Art of Clinical Care*. New York: Raven Press.

Scherer, K.R. (1981) 'Speech and emotional states.' In J.K. Darby (ed) *Speech Evaluation in Psychiatry*. New York: Grune and Stratton.

Scherer, K.R. (1986) 'Vocal affect expression: A review and model for further research.' *Psychological Bulletin 99*. 143–165.

Sheridan, M.D. (1975) *Children's Developmental Progress*. Windsor: NFER Publishing.

Shimoda, T.A. (1994) *'Excellent communication skills required' for Engineering Managers*. New York: American Society of Civil Engineers.

Siegman, A.W. (1987) 'The telltale voice: Nonverbal messages of verbal communication.' In A.W. Siegman and S. Feldstein, *Nonverbal Behavior and Communication*, (2nd edition). New Jersey: Lawrence Erlbaum Associates.

Spiegel, J. and Machotka, P. (1974) *Messages of the Body*. New York: Free Press.

Stewart, C.J. and Cash, W.B. (1988) *Interviewing: Principles and Practices*, (5th edition). Iowa: W.C. Brown.

The 3M Meeting Management Team (1994) *Mastering Meetings*. London: McGraw-Hill.

Thompson, J. (1984) 'Communicating with patients.' In R. Fitzpatrick, J. Hinton, S. Newman, G. Scambler and J. Thompson (eds) *The Experience of Illness*. London: Tavistock.

Thompson, J., Newell, R. and Dryden, W. (1991) 'Clinical Problems: An introduction to the cognitive-behavioural approach.' In W. Dryden and R.

Rentoul (eds) *Clinical Problems: A Cognitive-behavioural Approach.* London: Routledge.

Trower, P., Bryant, B. and Argyle, M. (1978) *Social Skills and Mental Health.* London: Methuen.

Watson, O.M. (1970) *Proxemic Behaviour: A Cross Cultural Study.* The Hague: Mouton.

Waxer, P.H. (1974) 'Non-verbal cues for depression.' *Journal of Abnormal Psychology 83,* 319–322.

Wilder, C. (1990) *The Presentations Kit.* New York: John Wiley and Sons.

Wilkinson, J. and Canter, S. (1982) *Social Skills Training Manual.* London: Wiley and Sons.

Wilson-Barnett, J. (1991) 'Providing relevant information for patients and their families.' In R. Corney, *Developing Communication and Counselling Skills in Medicine.* London: Routledge.

Woodall, W.G. and Burgoon, J.K. (1981) 'The effects of nonverbal synchrony on message comprehension and persuasiveness.' *Journal of Non-Verbal Behaviour 5,* 207–223.

Zahn, G.L. (1991) 'Face-to-face communication in an office setting: The effects of position, proximity and exposure.' *Communication Research 18,* 737–754.

Zaidel, S.F. and Mehrabian, A. (1969) 'The ability to communicate and infer positive and negative attitudes facially and vocally.' *Journal of Experimental Research in Personality 3,* 233–241.

Subject Index

adult case history, 95–99
agenda,
   circulating, 177, 185
   example, 185
   setting the agenda for
     a meeting, 183–5
aggressive clients, 109–10
aides-memoire, 248–9
ambiguity, 59, 280
angry clients, 109
application forms, 150
applying for a post, 143
   appearance, 150–2
   feedback from
     interview, 154
   interview, 152–4
   references, 150
   see also curriculum
     vitae, and
     application forms
appraisal
   definition, 118
   evaluation of appraiser,
     126–7
   improving appraisal
     systems, 125–6
   preparation, 119–20,
     121, 124,
     127–31
   process of appraisal,
     119–20

purpose of an appraisal
   system, 118
role of the appraisee,
   124–5
role of the appraiser,
   121–3
articulation, 259, 263
articulatory awareness
   exercises, 276–7
attention curve, 246
attention domains, 91
audience
   engaging, 288–9
   feedback, 290, 295
   participation, 289
   researching, 239–40,
     335, 336
audio playback, 301,
   303, 304, 314
audio tapes, 310
audio-visual aids
   benefits, 246–7
   choosing, 301, 304

bar charts, 359–63
behavioural rehearsal,
   328, 329, 330
bodily contact see touch
body posture see posture
brainstorming, 242–3,
   324–5, 327
breathing, 256–7,
   261–2, 274, 275
British Sign Language,
   80–1
business meeting
   definition, 208
   purpose, 208–9

case conference, 223–4
case history, 86, 92, 93,
   94–95
chairing
   committee meetings,
     227
   controlling difficult
     members, 188–9
   encouraging
     participation, 187
   evaluating your skills,
     198–9
   opening the meeting,
     186–7
clarity, 19, 263, 281
clients with a
   communication
   difficulty,
   comprehension
     problems, 111–12
   general guidelines, 111
   hearing loss, 80,
     113–14
   identifying, 110
   unclear speech, 111
clinical interviews
   asking questions, 92–3
   checking on accuracy,
     93–4
   closure, 115
   establishing rapport, 89
   giving advice, 107–8
   giving information,
     105–7
   improving memory
     and
     understanding,
     106–7
   introductions, 90
   listening, 91–2
   maintaining control, 93
   note taking, 114
   preparation, 86–7

questions, 92–3
seating, 87–9
setting an agenda, 90
structure, 92
clinic room, 88–9
committees
    ad hoc or special
        committee, 227
    advisory committee,
        227
    constitution, 225
    definition, 225
    executive committee,
        227
    procedures, 229
    joint committee, 227
    selecting committee
        members, 227
    standing committee,
        226
    sub committee, 227
contact culture, 7
conversational oil, 20
coping mechanisms,
    69–70, 72
curriculum vitae
    chronological, 145–7
    functional, 148–9
    trainee or graduate
        entry, 147–8
    writing a CV 143–5,
        150

deaf/blind clients, 80, 82
deaf/blind manual
    alphabet, 82
deaf clients, 80, 112
dealing with criticism,
    109, 124–5
delegate, 228–9
demonstrations, 325–6
diagnosis, 105

diaphragm, 255, 256,
    257, 261, 262, 275
disciplinary
    definition, 159
    interviewee 162–3
    interviewer 163–4
    organising the
        interview, 161
    preparation, 160–1
    venue, 160
distressed clients, 108–9
drawings, 309

empathy, 90–1
explanations
    analogies, 342–3
    anecdotes, 343
    examples, 342
    improving, 342
    quotes, 343
    types of, 59–60
eye-contact
    definition, 9
    interviews, 46
    presentations, 24,
        288–9, 294–5,
        355
    role of, 9–10

facial expression
    definition, 10
    role of, 11–12
    interviews, 46
    presentations, 290, 295
finger spelling, 81
flip chart, 297, 301, 302,
    304, 312
fundamental frequency,
    258

gaze see eye-contact
gesture
    definition, 12
    types of, 12–14
    presentations, 295–6,
        298
getting feedback, 25,
    60–1, 154
getting into role, 329–30
giving advice, 107–8
giving bad news, 106
giving feedback, 330–1
giving information
    appropriate language,
        57
    emphasising, 59
    explicit categorisation,
        106–7
    information, 55
    ordering information,
        58
    selecting key points,
        58, 105
grievance interviews
    definition, 159
    interviewee, 161–2
    interviewer, 162
    organising, 161
    preparation, 160–1
    venue, 160

hand-outs, 285–6
hard-of-hearing clients,
    81, 112–14
head and neck exercises,
    273–4
head movements, 15–16
hesitations, 281
horizontal bar charts,
    360–1
how a sound is made,
    254–5

ideographs, 13
image, 152, 169–70, 204
interpreters
  booking an interpreter,
    84–5
  communication
    context, 78
  definition, 76
  guidelines for working
    with an
    interpreter, 79–80
  reasons for, 75
  responsibilities, 77–8
  role, 76
interpreters for the
    sensory impaired
  definition, 80
  manual language
    interpreter, 83
  sign interpreters, 82–3
  working with, 82
interviews in general
  asking questions,
    49–51
  checking
    understanding, 65
  encouraging
    contributions
    from the
    interviewee, 51–2
  introductions, 38–9
  maintaining control, 52
  preparation, 36
  purpose, 33
  recording information,
    52
  setting an agenda, 39
  setting up the room,
    35–6
  structure of interviews,
    33
  structuring
    questioning, 50–1

time boundaries, 37, 64
interview rooms, 35
interviewer bias, 45, 47
intonation, 18–19, 258,
    264, 277–9

job description, 134–5
job information package,
    136–7
job specification, 135–6

language
  content, 21
  form, 22
  structure, 22
  use, 23
  vocabulary, 58, 107,
    280, 282
leakage, 13
lectures
  active study, 340
  explaining, 342–3
  evaluation, 343–9
  making your lecture
    interesting, 341–2
  preparation, 339
  structure, 340–1
line graphs, 364
lip speakers, 81
listener
  a good listener, 24
  appreciation of, 25
  attending behaviour,
    10, 11, 15, 16
listening
  active listening, 341
  attention domains, 91
  effective listening,
    46–49
  factors affecting, 55–7

improving memory
  and
    understanding of
    information, 106
lungs, 255–6, 257, 258,
    262

media interviews
  body language, 168
  group interviews,
    168–9
  image, 169–70
  preparation, 167
medical terminology or
    jargon, 57, 107,
    335, 337
meetings,
  evaluating
    effectiveness,
    209–10
  large, 209
  membership, 176–7,
    209
  reasons for, 208–9
  small, 209
  time-tabling, 176
meeting members
  contributing, 196–7
  good meeting
    members, 189
  listening, 190, 191,
    200, 205–6,
    224, 234
  organisation, 194
  preparation, 195
meeting member's
    checklist, 211
meetings rooms
  access, 179
  acoustics, 179
  booking 180
  catering 179

decor 179
facilities, 178
lighting, 178
location, 177
preparation, 180
room set-up, 178
seating, 178
shape, 178
size, 178
temperature, 179
meetings secretary, 190–4
minutes,
    example, 193
    reasons for, 191
    recording, 190–1
    writing, 191–2
mixed messages, 295
modelling, 327
models, 301, 305, 315
multi-disciplinary teams,
    213
    see also teams
multi-media, 301, 304,
    305, 315
multiple bar charts, 361

nerves, 70, 205, 207,
    295, 296, 298,
    336–7
non-contact culture, 7
non-verbal
    communication, 4,
    72, 90, 114, 153,
    285, 294
note takers, 81

observation, 45–6
open body position, 15,
    90, 168, 355

overhead projector, 301,
    302, 304, 313–14

pace, 56, 78, 161, 247,
    260, 263–4, 267,
    282–3, 290
    see also rate of speech
paediatric case history,
    100–4
paralinguistic features of
    communication, 5,
    17–20, 72, 109
partially hearing clients,
    81, 112
pauses, 10, 51, 53, 72,
    122, 253, 267,
    282, 283
personal space, 6
pictographs, 13
pie charts, 363
pointing, 13
position, 88–9, 196,
    297–8
position for exercising,
    269–70
posters, 327
posture,
    definition, 12, 14
    interviews, 46, 90,
        153, 168
    meetings, 196, 205
    presentations, 295,
        296–7
    role of, 14–15, 16
    see also open body
        positions
posture and breathing,
    261–2
posture and relaxation,
    260, 267, 269
preparing visuals, 364–5

presentations,
    aides-memoire, 248–9
    attention gaining
        devices, 246
    dealing with questions,
        283–5
    final dress rehearsal,
        249
    finishing, 248, 291,
        356, 358
    introductions, 288,
        354, 357–8
    planning, 241–4
    preparation, 239–41
    structure, 244–5
    time factors, 247–8,
        291, 321–2
problem solving, 123,
    232–3, 326–7
prognosis, 56, 106
proportional bar charts,
    361–3
proximity, 6–7

questions
    broad, 50, 51
    clarification, 49, 94
    closed, 49, 50, 51, 52,
        93
    forced alternative, 43
    leading, 50, 93, 139
    multiple, 49
    multiple-choice, 43
    open questions, 49,
        50, 51, 92, 122,
        123, 139, 187,
        344
    specific questions, 50,
        51
    wh- type questions,
        42–3
questionnaires, 42–3, 45

quotes, 343

rate of speech, 18, 19, 264, 283
realia (real objects), 301, 304, 305, 315
recruitment interviews
  asking questions, 140
  evaluating the candidate, 141
  formal interviews, 138
  informal interviews, 138–9
  introductions, 140
  organisation, 138
  panel, 138, 139
  preparing questions, 139–40
  providing feedback to the candidate, 141
  recording information, 141
relaxation, 15, 260–1, 263, 267, 269
relaxation exercises, 207, 270–3
reflecting, 91, 190
representative, 229
research, 357
  content of presentation, 358
  displaying numerical information, 308–9, 358–64
  presentation checklist, 366–7
resonance, 17, 259, 263
resonance exercises, 275–6

resonating cavities, 256, 258, 263
rhythm of speech, 13, 19, 112, 263, 264, 283
role play, 328–30

safety hints for audio visual aids, 311
self-touching actions, 14
selling your service
  describing your service, 352–3
  persuading the purchaser, 353
  researching your buyer, 353
  your message, 355
signs supporting English, 80, 81
silences *see* pauses
slide projector, 297, 301, 302–3, 304, 312–13
smiling, 11
  see also facial expression
speech sounds, 22–3, 259, 263, 276
style or register, 23–4
summaries
  definition, 65
  interviews 52, 61, 64, 94, 115, 123, 162
  meetings, 190, 192, 223
  practical exercise, 67
  presentations, 244, 291, 341

tables, 359
teams
  avoiding conflict, 216–18
  characteristics of a successful team, 221
  establishing roles, 214, 218–20
  leading a team, 215–16
  participation, 218
  rewards, 213–14
  team building, 214–15
  team, definition, 213
team presentations
  audio-visual aids, 355
  organisation, 353–4
text on visuals, 246–7, 305–6, 309, 310, 312, 365
touch, 7–9, 14, 109, 153
use of colour in visuals, 306–8, 309, 355, 361, 362, 363, 364, 365
using appropriate language, 57, 107, 280, 335
vertical bar charts, 359–60
video playback, 301, 303, 304, 314
video tapes, 311
visualisation, 272–3
vocal folds, 255, 256, 257–8, 259, 263, 275
vocal tract, 256, 258, 259, 263
voice
  audibility, 261, 262
  care of, 266–8

as a performance tool,
        260, 264
    pitch, 18, 19, 253,
        254, 258, 277
    projection, 262–3
    tone of voice, 19, 90,
        162, 168, 253,
        258, 278–9
    voice quality, 17, 19,
        266
    volume, 17–18, 19,
        253, 261, 262,
        264, 267
vocal qualities, 25
waiting room, 87
warm-up activities, 324
whiteboard, 297, 301,
        304, 312
working party
    definition, 232
    membership, 232
    participation, 233–4
    problem solving,
        232–3
workshops
    accommodation
        319–20
    activities, 324–8
    audio-visual aids,
        320–1
    benefits, 319
    format, 321
    manual, 322–3
    organising activities,
        323–4
    planning, 321–2
    seating, 320

Author
Index

Anstey, E. 229
Argyle, M. 9, 12, 13, 14, 15, 19, 295
Armstrong, S.L. 19, 283
Aronson, A.E. 12
Arvey, R. 153
Atherton, S.T. 106

Baken, R.J. 256, 258
Bales, R.F. 196
Berne, E. 163
Binstead, D. 330
Bird, J. 92
Bligh, D. 246
Bond, T. 323
Borden, G.J. 254, 256
Boydell, T. 135, 141
Bradshaw, P.W. 106
Breakwell, G.M. 167, 169
Brown, G. 59, 281, 342
Brown, J.R. 12
Bryant, B. 14, 295
Bull, P. 13, 15, 16
Bunch, M. 247, 256, 268
Burgoon, J.K. 295
Burgoyne, J. 135, 141
Burnard, P. 91
Butler, P.E. 124

Campion, J. 153
Canter, S. 14
Cash, W.B. 65
Citrenbaum, C. 59
Clare, A. 87, 89
Cohen, W.I. 95
Cohen-Cole, S.A. 92
Connelly, G. 13
Cook, M. 9, 88
Corney, R. 57
Croner 122, 162

Darly, F.L. 12
Dean, J. 9
Denes, P.B. 258
Deuchar, M. 81
Dickson, A. 124, 125
Dickson, D.A. 61, 66, 69
Downs, M.P. 12
Dryden, W. 45
Duncan, S. 15

Ekman, P. 11, 12, 13
Ellis, R. 341

Fawcus, R. 258
Fiske, D.W. 15
Forsyth, P. 282, 290
Freeburn, R. 196, 283, 290
Freedman, N. 14
Frick, R.W. 18
Friedrich, G. 15
Friesen, W.V. 11, 12, 13

Gahagan, J. 10
Gask, L. 90
Gibbs, G. 339, 246, 341
Gilroy, J. 12
Gimson, A.C. 18
Goodworth, C.T. 138, 150
Graham, J. 295
Gratus, J. 208

Habeshaw, S. 341
Habeshaw, T. 341
Hall, E.T. 6
Hampton, J.R. 93
Hargie, O. 61, 66, 69
Harrigan, J.A. 90
Harris, K.S. 254, 256
Harrison, M.J.E. 93
Hart, R. 15
Hauge, M. 241
Havelock, P. 92
Herriot, P. 141
Heylin, A. 154, 168, 205, 353
Hirano, M. 253
Hoffman, S.P. 14
Holliday, P.L. 12
Hunt, N. 122, 125
Huntington, D. 90

Ingram, I.M. 14
Izard, C.E. 11, 16, 196

Jay, A. 313
Jourard, S.M. 7

Kaplan, H.M. 255
Kent, R.D. 257, 258
Kincey, J.A. 106
King, M. 59
Kleinke, C.L. 10
Knapp, M.L. 15
Koontz, H. 123
Krasner, L. 15

Lamb, W. 12, 14, 15
L'Armand, K. 10
Ley, P. 55, 105, 106
Locke, M. 225

Machotka, P. 16
Maddux, R.B. 118, 122
Maguire, P. 106, 109
Martin, S. 256
Matarazzo, J.D. 51
McClintock, A. 341
Mehrabian, A. 15, 295
Messer, D.J. 13
Mitchell, J.R.A. 93
Morris, D. 12, 13
Morrow, N.C. 69
Mowbray, R.M. 14
Murphy, C.M. 13
Myerscough, P.R. 93

Newell, R. 45, 90
Northern, J.L. 12
Novik, L. 59

O'Donnell, C. 123
Open University 326
Øvretveit, 351, 352
Oxman, T.E. 90

Packard, P. 118
Pedler, M. 135, 141
Pendleton, D. 92
Perkins, W.H. 257, 258
Pinson, E.N. 258
Porritt, L. 90
Pritchard, J.S. 93

Randall, G. 353
Randell, G. 118
Rees, W.D. 57
Riseborough, M.G. 295
Roberts, C. 153
Rogers, W. 295
Rosenshine, B. 264
Rosenthal, R. 90

Saslow, G. 51
Saunders, C. 61, 66
Scherer, K.R. 18
Schofield, T. 92
Schulman, G. 15
Seymour, C. 93
Sheridan, M.D. 11
Shimoda, T.A. 58, 290
Siegman, A.W. 18
Slater, J. 118
Spiegel, J. 16
Stewart, C.J. 65

Tate, P. 92
The 3-M Meeting
    Management Team,
    208, 247
Thompson, J. 45, 89
Timbury, G.C. 14
Trower, P. 14, 295

Watson, E. 12, 14, 15
Watson, O.M. 10
Waxer, P.H. 16
Wiens, A.N. 51
Wilder, C. 244, 354
Wilkinson, J. 14
Wilson-Barnett, J. 105
Woodall, W.G. 295

Zahn, G.L. 6

Zaidel, S.F. 295